CONTROLLING YOUR KIDNEY HEALTH

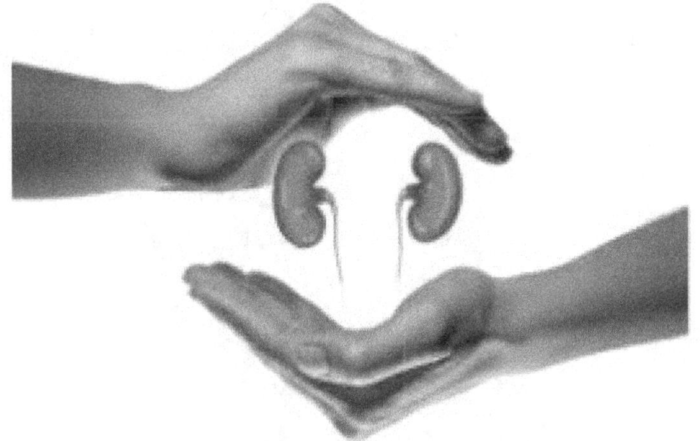

The All-Inclusive Handbook to Optimize Your Kidneys and Live Better

Dr Heather Perry MD

No part of this publication may be reproduced, distributed, or transmitted in any form or by any means, including photocopying, recording, or other electronic or mechanical methods without the prior written permission of the author, except in the case of brief quotations embodied in critical reviews and certain other noncommercial uses permitted by copyright law.

Copyright © Dr Heather Perry MD 2023

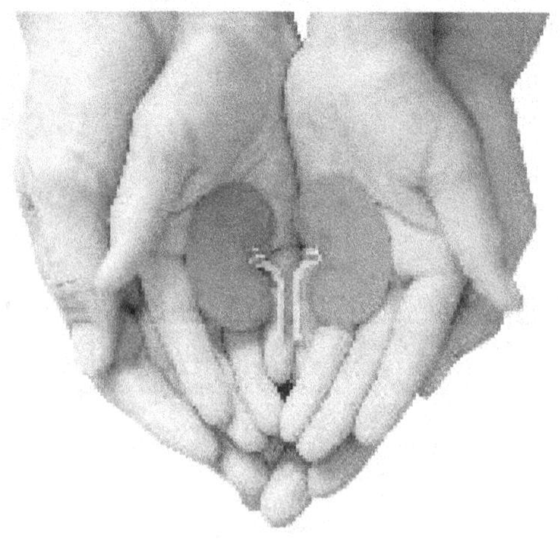

Table Of Contents

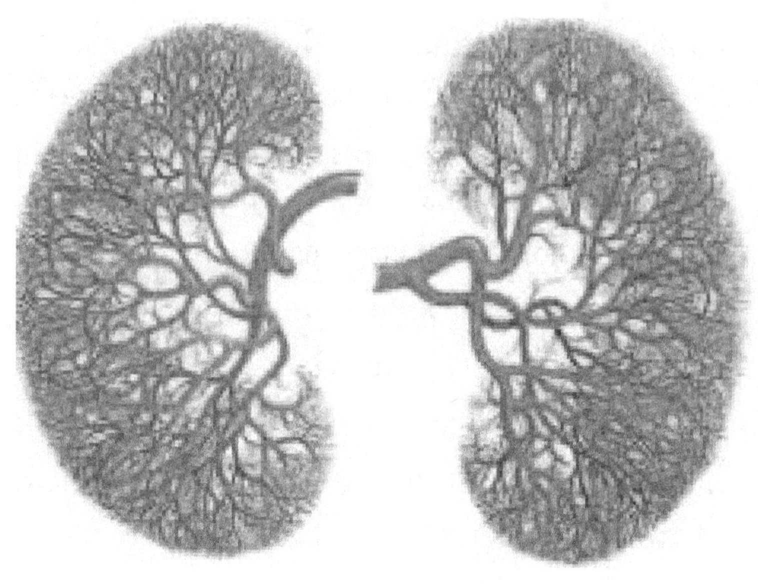

Chapter 1: Introduction

Imagine waking up in the morning with a sense of dread in every single day. The same things must be done each and every morning: wake up, take your medicine, make yourself stick to a restricted diet, and drive yourself to the dialysis clinic. Since your kidneys are no longer able to function properly, you will have to spend many hours there hooked up to a machine that will filter your blood. You do your best to ignore the exhaustion, the nausea, and the overpowering feeling that there is no hope at all at this time.

This was the truth that I faced. I disregarded the warning signals of renal illness, which included chronic weariness, edema in my legs, and unquenchable thirst. As a result, I was diagnosed with kidney disease some years ago. But finally, my symptoms reached a point where they could no longer be ignored, and I was eventually given a diagnosis of stage 4 renal disease. My medical team informed me that a kidney transplant was probably going to be necessary for me, but that I would have to wait for a donor. Dialysis was the only choice I had available to me in the meanwhile.

My life turned into a monotonous routine of trips to the doctor, dialysis treatments, and taking drugs. I was unable to do my job duties, and I struggled to muster the strength to even leave the home. I felt like I was being held back by a body that was failing me, while at the same time I watched my friends and relatives go on with their lives.

Yet, after that, a shift occurred. I was relieved to learn that there was a chance that my kidney condition may be reversed with various lifestyle adjustments, dietary alterations, and alternative treatments. I started doing some research and experimenting with various ways, and I saw that I was gradually beginning to feel better as a result. My level of energy rose, my appetite became better, and I experienced a general improvement in my feeling of well-being.

Now, I am here to testify that it is really possible to reverse renal illness. I am no longer dependent on dialysis, and I have been able to avoid the need of receiving a transplant. Instead, I am now leading a rich and busy life, during which I take delight in the straightforward luxuries that were before out of my grasp. My trip was not without its challenges, but in the end, it was well worth it. And at this point, I feel obligated to pass on what I've learned to those who could be afflicted with renal illness.

What is kidney disease?

Kidney disease is a condition that affects the functioning of the kidneys, which are essential organs responsible for filtering waste and excess fluids from the blood, regulating blood pressure, and producing hormones that help to maintain healthy bone density and red blood cell production.

Kidney disease can be broadly classified into two main types: acute kidney injury (AKI) and chronic kidney disease (CKD). AKI is a sudden and usually reversible loss of kidney function that occurs over a short period of time, while CKD is a progressive and usually irreversible decline in kidney function that occurs over a period of months or years.

CKD is further categorized into five stages based on the estimated glomerular filtration rate (eGFR) which measures how well the kidneys are filtering the blood. The stages range from Stage 1 (eGFR >90) to Stage 5 (eGFR <15), which is known as end-stage renal disease (ESRD).

The most common causes of CKD include diabetes, high blood pressure, glomerulonephritis (inflammation of the kidney's filtering units), and polycystic kidney disease (an inherited disorder that causes the growth of cysts in the kidneys).

Symptoms of kidney disease can vary depending on the stage and underlying cause of the disease. In the early stages of CKD, patients may not have any symptoms at all, while in later stages, patients may experience fatigue, fluid retention, difficulty sleeping, muscle cramps, and changes in urine output, color or smell.

Diagnosis of kidney disease involves a series of tests including blood tests, urine tests, and imaging studies. These tests can help to determine the level of kidney function and identify any underlying conditions that may be contributing to the disease.

Treatment for kidney disease varies depending on the stage and cause of the disease. In the early stages of CKD, lifestyle modifications such as exercise, weight loss, and dietary changes can be effective in slowing the progression of the disease. As CKD progresses, medications such as blood pressure-lowering drugs and erythropoietin-stimulating agents may be prescribed to manage symptoms and complications. In some cases, dialysis or kidney transplant may be necessary to replace the function of the failing kidneys.

Overall, early diagnosis and management of kidney disease is critical for improving outcomes and preventing complications. Regular monitoring and follow-up with a healthcare provider is important for patients with kidney disease, even if they are not experiencing any symptoms.

Causes of kidney disease

There are several causes of kidney disease, ranging from genetic factors to lifestyle habits.

Here is a detailed overview of some of the most common causes:

- Diabetes: Diabetes is a chronic condition that affects the body's ability to produce or use insulin, leading to high levels of sugar (glucose) in the blood. Over time, high blood sugar can damage the tiny blood vessels in the kidneys, reducing their ability to filter waste from the blood. This can lead to a condition known as diabetic nephropathy, which is one of the leading causes of chronic kidney disease (CKD).

- High blood pressure: High blood pressure (hypertension) is a common condition that can damage the blood vessels in the kidneys, reducing their ability to filter waste and excess fluid from the blood. This can lead to CKD, and over time, can progress to end-stage renal disease (ESRD) that requires dialysis or kidney transplant.

- Glomerulonephritis: Glomerulonephritis is a condition in which the tiny filtering units in the kidneys, known as glomeruli, become inflamed and damaged. This can occur as a result of an infection, autoimmune disease, or other underlying condition. Glomerulonephritis can lead to CKD if not treated promptly.

- Polycystic kidney disease: Polycystic kidney disease (PKD) is a genetic disorder in which cysts grow in the kidneys, gradually replacing healthy tissue and impairing kidney function. PKD can lead to ESRD, and there is currently no cure for the condition.

- Urinary tract obstruction: Urinary tract obstruction occurs when something blocks the normal flow of urine from the kidneys to the bladder. This can occur due to a physical blockage, such as a kidney stone, or as a result of an underlying condition, such as an enlarged prostate. If left untreated, urinary tract obstruction can lead to kidney damage and CKD.

- Overuse of painkillers: Long-term use of certain painkillers, such as nonsteroidal anti-inflammatory drugs (NSAIDs), can damage the kidneys and lead to CKD. This is because these drugs can reduce blood flow to the kidneys, leading to reduced kidney function over time.

- Other factors: Other factors that can contribute to kidney disease include smoking, obesity, a family history of kidney disease, and certain infections or autoimmune diseases.

In summary, kidney disease can be caused by a wide range of factors, including genetic conditions, lifestyle habits, and underlying medical conditions. Early diagnosis and management of these underlying causes is critical for preventing kidney damage and slowing the progression of the disease.

Importance of early detection and treatment

Early detection and treatment of kidney disease is critical for preserving kidney function, preventing complications, and improving overall health outcomes. In this article, we will explore the importance of early detection and treatment of kidney disease, as well as some of the key strategies that can be used to achieve these goals.

Kidney disease is a silent killer that often goes unnoticed until it has progressed to an advanced stage. According to the National Kidney Foundation, approximately 37 million people in the United States have kidney disease, and most of them are not aware of it. This is because kidney disease often has no symptoms in its early stages, and by the time symptoms do appear, significant kidney damage may have already occurred.

Early detection of kidney disease is important because it allows healthcare providers to intervene early and prevent further damage to the kidneys. Early treatment can slow or even halt the progression of kidney disease, preventing the need for dialysis or kidney transplant later on.

Early detection and treatment of kidney disease can also prevent complications and improve overall health outcomes. Kidney disease can lead to a range of complications, including high blood pressure, anemia, bone disease, and heart disease. By detecting kidney disease early and treating it promptly, these complications can be prevented or managed effectively, improving quality of life and reducing the risk of premature death.

There are several strategies that can be used to achieve early detection and treatment of kidney disease. Here are some of the key approaches:

- Regular screening: Regular screening for kidney disease is essential for early detection. This involves a simple blood test to measure the level of creatinine in the blood, as well as a urine test to check for the presence of protein. These tests can help identify kidney disease in its early stages, when it is most treatable.

- Managing underlying conditions: Many underlying medical conditions can contribute to kidney disease, including diabetes, high blood pressure, and autoimmune diseases. Managing these conditions effectively can help prevent or slow the progression of kidney disease.

- Lifestyle modifications: Making lifestyle modifications, such as quitting smoking, eating a healthy diet, exercising regularly, and managing stress, can help prevent kidney disease and improve kidney function in those who have already been diagnosed.

- Medications: There are several medications that can be used to treat kidney disease and prevent complications. These may include medications to control blood pressure, reduce inflammation, or treat underlying conditions such as diabetes or autoimmune disease.

- Referral to a nephrologist: Referral to a nephrologist, or kidney specialist, can be helpful for managing more advanced cases of kidney disease. Nephrologists can provide specialized care and treatment, including dialysis and kidney transplant, when needed.

In conclusion, early detection and treatment of kidney disease is critical for preserving kidney function, preventing complications, and improving overall health outcomes. Regular screening, managing underlying conditions, making lifestyle modifications, using medications, and seeking care from a kidney specialist can all help achieve these goals. By taking a proactive approach to kidney health, individuals can reduce their risk of developing kidney disease and improve their overall quality of life.

The goal of reversing kidney disease

The restoration of kidney function and an improvement in the patient's overall health are the two primary objectives in the treatment of renal disease. It may be difficult to reverse renal disease since patients often need to make major adjustments to their lifestyle, undergo medical treatments, and be closely monitored by healthcare specialists.

The strategy that will be used to reverse renal disease will be determined by the underlying cause of the illness. For instance, if the kidney disease is brought on by diabetes or high blood pressure, then managing these underlying illnesses will be an important part of the treatment plan. Alterations to one's lifestyle, such as adopting a healthier diet, maintaining a regular exercise routine, and giving up smoking, could also be suggested.

Managing the underlying issues that cause kidney disease and making changes to one's way of life aren't the only things that can be done to reverse renal disease; there are also various medical therapies that may be employed. Medication to manage blood pressure, decrease inflammation, or treat diseases that lie deeper in the body may fall into this category. Dialysis or a kidney transplant may be required in some circumstances in order to restore normal kidney function.

It is essential to keep in mind that reversing renal disease is not always achievable, especially if the illness has proceeded to a more advanced level. In these situations, the objective of therapy will not be to completely cure the condition but rather to slow down or stop the advancement of the disease and avoid any consequences that may arise as a result of it.

Early identification and treatment of renal illness is critical for avoiding additional damage to the kidneys and maintaining kidney function. This is true even if the disease is already in an advanced state. Individuals who have kidney disease may enhance their chances of achieving these objectives and improving their outcomes by undergoing routine screenings, treating any underlying illnesses, modifying their lifestyles, taking prescribed medicines, and seeking out the treatment of a renal specialist.

Chapter 2: Understanding the Kidneys

Anatomy and physiology of the kidneys

The kidneys are a pair of bean-shaped organs that may be found in the lower back, one on each side of the spine. They are a component of the urinary system and play an important function in the regulation of blood pressure, the maintenance of the correct fluid and electrolyte balance, and the elimination of waste products from the body.

The cortex, the medulla, and the pelvis are the three primary components that make up each kidney. Nephrons are very small filtering units that are found in the millions in the cortex of the kidney, which is the outermost layer of the organ. The medulla is the most innermost portion of the kidney, and it is composed of structures known as renal pyramids. These renal pyramids are in charge of collecting urine. Urine is collected from the renal pyramids and directed into the pelvis, which is a hollow chamber located in the middle of the kidney. Urine is then transported to the bladder through the ureter, which connects to the bladder.

The nephron is the functional unit of the kidney and is responsible for filtering waste items out of the blood and creating urine. Nephrons also play a role in the production of tubules and collecting ducts. Each nephron is made up of a glomerulus, which is a collection of very small blood arteries, and a tubule, which is a long, winding structure that gathers and processes the filtered fluid. The glomerulus is the most prominent part of the nephron. As blood passes through the glomerulus, waste materials and fluids that are in excess are removed by the filtering process and collected in the tubule. After this, part of the fluid that has been filtered is reabsorbed by the tubule, and it is returned to the circulation. The remaining waste items are then expelled into the urine.

In addition, the kidneys are in charge of maintaining the correct fluid and electrolyte balance throughout the body. This is made possible by a sophisticated network of interactions between hormones and enzymes, which regulates the quantity of fluid and electrolytes that are stored in the body as opposed to being passed out in the urine. For example, the hormone aldosterone encourages the retention of salt and water in the body, while the hormone antidiuretic hormone (ADH) encourages the reabsorption of water in the kidneys. Both of these hormones are produced by the pituitary gland.

The kidneys are responsible for a number of important bodily functions, including maintaining a healthy balance of fluids and electrolytes, as well as controlling blood pressure. Renin is a hormone that is produced by the kidneys, and it plays a role in the regulation of blood pressure by either narrowing or widening the blood vessels. When blood pressure is too low, the kidneys secrete an enzyme called renin, which kicks off a chain of chemical processes that causes blood vessels to narrow and, as a result, raises blood pressure. If a person has high blood pressure, their kidneys will produce less renin, which will cause their blood vessels to expand and ultimately result in reduced blood pressure.

In general, the structure and physiology of the kidneys are intricate and carefully controlled, which is a reflection of the significant function that these organs play in the preservation of overall health and wellbeing. It is essential for healthcare providers who are working to prevent, diagnose, and treat kidney disease, as well as for individuals who are seeking to maintain optimal kidney health throughout their lives, to have a complete understanding of the structure and function of the kidneys. This is true for both individuals and for healthcare providers.

Functions of the kidneys

The kidneys are critical organs that are responsible for a variety of fundamental processes throughout the body. The following is a list of the major functions of the kidneys:

- The kidneys are responsible for a significant portion of the fluid and electrolyte regulation that occurs in the body. This is an extremely important function that the kidneys do. They do this by removing waste materials, surplus fluids, and electrolytes from the circulation and then excreting them in the urine, so regulating the amount and composition of the body's fluids.

- The kidneys are responsible for the removal of waste products by filtering them out of the blood and passing them out of the body in the urine. In addition to urea, creatinine, and uric acid, these waste products also include a variety of additional compounds that are harmful to the body.

- The kidneys are responsible for a significant portion of the regulatory work that goes into maintaining a healthy blood pressure. They generate hormones that contribute to the regulation of the amount of blood that is found inside the body as well as the narrowing and widening of blood vessels.

- The production of erythropoietin The kidneys are responsible for the synthesis of a hormone known as erythropoietin. This hormone encourages the formation of red blood cells in the bone marrow.

- Activation of vitamin D The kidneys are responsible for a significant portion of the activation of vitamin D, which is essential for the body to have in order to absorb calcium and to keep its bones and teeth in good condition.

- The kidneys play a role in the regulation of the acid-base balance by excreting excess acids or bases into urine, which in turn helps to keep the pH level of the blood at a stable level.

- The kidneys have a part to play in the process of keeping the body's fluid balance in check when the body is exerting itself via physical activity. By preserving both water and electrolytes, they contribute to the regulation of the quantity of fluid that is lost due to perspiration.

The kidneys, as a whole, are responsible for performing crucial processes that are necessary for the upkeep of general health and fitness. A variety of health issues, such as abnormalities in fluid and electrolyte levels, high blood pressure, anemia, and diseases of the bones, may be brought on by dysfunction in the kidneys. For the sake of one's long-term health and well-being, it is very necessary to ensure that optimum kidney function is preserved via the adoption of good lifestyle practices, the performance of routine screenings, and the prompt diagnosis and treatment of renal disease.

How the kidneys filter waste from the blood

A complicated process that takes place over the course of many stages, the kidneys remove waste products from the blood.

- The first phase in the process is called glomerular filtration, and it takes place in the renal corpuscles that are located in the cortex of the kidney. At this point, waste materials and excess fluids in the circulation are separated from the rest of the blood by passing it through a network of capillaries known as the glomerulus. This network functions like a sieve. After being cleansed, the blood is transported into the renal tubules.

- Tubular reabsorption: The renal tubules, in the subsequent process known as tubular reabsorption, reabsorb part of the filtered fluids and electrolytes, such as sodium, potassium, and chloride, that are necessary for the body to maintain its equilibrium. This phase helps to ensure that the body does not lose an excessive amount of components that are vital to its functioning.

- The last stage is called tubular secretion, and it is performed by the renal tubules. During this step, the renal tubules produce waste materials like urea and creatinine that were not removed by the filtration process in the step before it. At this stage, the kidneys are given the opportunity to purge the body of any waste products that may still be present while also ensuring that the correct electrolyte balance is maintained.

Hormones such as aldosterone and antidiuretic hormone (ADH) are two examples of hormones that play a role in the regulation of the filtration process. These hormones contribute to the regulation of the quantity of fluid and electrolytes that are reabsorbed and released by the kidneys. In addition, the renal arteries provide a steady flow of blood to the kidneys, which enables the kidneys to filter waste items from the blood and maintain the general fluid and electrolyte balance of the body.

It is possible for the process of filtration to be disrupted if the kidneys become damaged or diseased. This may result in an accumulation of waste products in the blood and the development of a variety of health issues. It is essential to undergo routine screening tests in order to diagnose and treat renal disease in its earliest stages in order to preserve optimum kidney function and general health.

Common kidney diseases and their symptoms

There are many distinct forms of kidney illnesses, and each presents its own unique collection of signs and symptoms.

The following is a list of some of the most prevalent kidney illnesses and the symptoms that are linked with them:

- Chronic Kidney Disease (CKD) is a disorder that lasts for a lengthy period of time in which the kidneys progressively lose function during the course of their disease. A person who has this condition may have symptoms such as weariness, weakness, trouble sleeping, lack of appetite, nausea, and swelling in the legs and ankles.

- Acute kidney injury, often known as AKI, is a rapid and transient reduction in the function of the kidneys. A reduction in the amount of urine that is passed, retention of fluid, weariness, disorientation, and chest discomfort are all possible symptoms.

- Glomerulonephritis is a kind of kidney illness that is characterized by inflammation of the glomeruli, which are the very small filters that are found inside the kidneys. In addition to swelling in the legs and ankles, symptoms may include blood in the urine, high blood pressure, protein in the urine, and elevated blood pressure.

- Stones in the kidneys are hard deposits that may cause excruciating discomfort as they move through the urinary system. Stones in the kidneys are formed when urine contains crystals. Intense pain in the back, side, or groin, nausea and vomiting, and blood in the urine are some of the symptoms that may be experienced.

- Polycystic Kidney Disease (PKD) is a hereditary illness in which cysts grow in the kidneys, causing them to expand and lose function over time. PKD is an abbreviation for polycystic kidney disease. Pain in the back or sides, elevated blood pressure, and the presence of blood in the urine are all possible symptoms.

- Nephrotic syndrome is a disorder in which the kidneys lose excessive quantities of protein into the urine. Nephrotic syndrome is also known as nephrotic syndrome. The swelling of the legs and ankles, weariness, lack of appetite, and frothy urine are some of the symptoms that may be experienced.

- Pyelonephritis is a form of kidney infection that may develop if bacteria from the bladder make their way up to the kidneys. This can cause a condition known as pyelonephritis. Fever, chills, nausea and vomiting, discomfort in the back or side, and frequent urination are some of the symptoms that may be experienced.

It is essential to keep in mind that the early stages of various kidney disorders may not be accompanied by any noticeable symptoms. It is essential to do blood and urine tests on a regular basis as part of a screening regimen in order to diagnose kidney disease at an early stage and maintain optimum kidney function in order to ward off long-term consequences. It is imperative that you get medical help as soon as possible if you suffer any of the symptoms that were listed above.

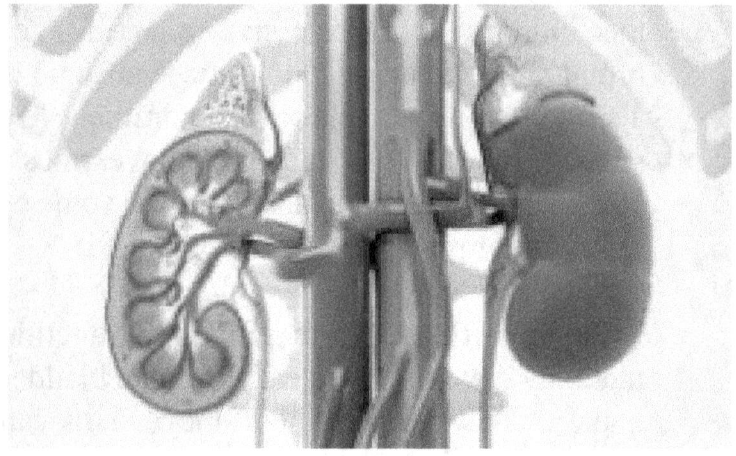

Chapter 3: Diagnosing Kidney Disease

Signs and symptoms of kidney disease

There is a vast variety of signs and symptoms associated with kidney illness, and they might change based on the kind of kidney disease and the stage it is in.

The following is a list of indications and symptoms of renal illness that are common:

- Fatigue is defined as the feeling of being weary and weak, even after getting adequate rest.

- Swelling may occur in the hands, face, feet, and legs as well as the ankles and feet. Edema is the medical term for this swelling, which develops when the kidneys are unable to clear extra fluid from the body as they normally would.

- Alterations in Urination These include changes in the amount, color, and frequency of your urine. This might include peeing more often, a reduction in the amount of urine that is produced, or urine that is bloody, frothy, or black in color.

- Trouble breathing or a shortness of breath is another name for shortness of breath. This condition may develop if renal dysfunction leads to an accumulation of extra fluid in the lungs.

- High Blood Pressure: High blood pressure that is not under control, which might cause more kidney damage.

- Nausea and Vomiting Nausea, vomiting, and a lack of appetite are all symptoms that may appear when there is an accumulation of waste materials in the blood.

- Cramps in the Muscles An electrolyte imbalance brought on by renal illness may bring on cramps in the muscles, particularly throughout the night.

- Itching: An accumulation of waste products in the blood may cause persistent itching as well as dry skin. [Cause and effect]

- Pain in the Bones Weakened bones, which are a side effect of renal illness, may lead to bone discomfort and even fractures.

It is essential to keep in mind that kidney disease may not present any symptoms in some people until the illness has proceeded to a more advanced state. For the purpose of avoiding complications and effectively treating renal disease, routine screening and early identification by blood and urine testing are both essential. It is essential that you see your healthcare provider if you are experiencing any of the aforementioned symptoms in order to identify the underlying reason and obtain the therapy that is suitable for your condition.

Blood tests to diagnose kidney disease

Diagnostic and monitoring procedures for renal illness often include blood testing.

The following is a list of common blood tests that are used to evaluate kidney function:

- Creatinine is a waste product that is created by muscles and then filtered out of the blood by the kidneys. The serum creatinine test measures the amount of creatinine in the blood. A test called a serum creatinine test analyzes the amount of creatinine that is present in the blood, which may provide insight into the health of the kidneys. Creatinine levels in the blood that are higher than normal are an indicator of impaired kidney function.

- The Blood Urea Nitrogen (BUN) Test: The BUN test measures a waste product called blood urea nitrogen, which is created by the liver and then removed from the blood by the kidneys. A blood urea nitrogen, or BUN, test determines the percentage of nitrogen in the blood that comes from urea. When measured in the blood, elevated levels of BUN may be an indicator of impaired kidney function.

- The term "estimated glomerular filtration rate" (eGFR) refers to a computation that attempts to determine how effectively the kidneys are removing waste materials from the blood. The estimated glomerular filtration rate (eGFR) of a person is determined by using their age, gender, race, and creatinine concentration. A reduced eGFR shows that kidney function is impaired.

- Electrolyte Levels Electrolytes are minerals that are necessary for the body to operate normally. Some examples of electrolytes are sodium, potassium, and calcium. Electrolyte imbalances are a common complication of renal illness, and they may manifest themselves in a broad variety of ways.

- A complete blood count, often known as a CBC, is a test that evaluates many aspects of the patient's blood, such as the number of red blood cells, white blood cells, and platelets. Anemia, infections, and bleeding problems may all be caused by kidney illness because it can interfere with the generation of these cells.

Blood tests like this may assist in the diagnosis of kidney disease as well as the monitoring of its development. In the event that you are having any symptoms or have any risk factors for kidney disease, it is imperative that you consult with your healthcare physician to evaluate whether or not blood tests are required.

Urine tests to diagnose kidney disease

Diagnostic and monitoring procedures for kidney disease often include testing urine. The following is a list of the most popular types of urine tests that are used to evaluate kidney function:

- Test for Urine Albumin: Albumin is a kind of protein that is often only detected in the blood and not in the urine. Urine Albumin Test A test that measures urine albumin may provide insight into the health of the kidneys by determining the amount of albumin that is present in the urine. A possible indicator of kidney injury is an increase in the amount of albumin found in the urine.

- Test for Urine Protein: A urine protein test is one that determines how much protein is present in the urine. In the same way that a high urine albumin level may signal kidney disease, so too can an elevated urine protein level.

- Test for Creatinine in the Urine: A test for creatinine in the urine measures the amount of creatinine that is present in the urine. In order to compute the estimated glomerular filtration rate (eGFR), which provides an indication of how well the kidneys are removing waste products from the blood, this test is often performed in conjunction with a serum creatinine test.

- Urinalysis: A urinalysis is an extensive test that investigates the chemical and physical components of the urine. Urinalysis is a test that may determine whether or not a person has kidney disease by determining whether or not the urine contains blood, protein, or other chemicals.

The kidney disease may be diagnosed and its development monitored with the use of these urine tests. In the event that you are having any symptoms or have any risk factors for kidney disease, it is imperative that you consult with your healthcare physician to evaluate whether or not urine testing are required.

Imaging tests to diagnose kidney disease

Imaging studies are often used both to identify renal disease and to track its progression. The following is a list of common imaging tests that are used to evaluate kidney function:

- An ultrasound is a diagnostic procedure that produces pictures of the kidneys by using sound waves of a very high frequency. This test may assist in determining whether or not the kidneys have been damaged, such as by the development of cysts or tumors, and it can also assist in determining the size and form of the kidneys.

- CT Scan: A CT scan is a diagnostic procedure that produces comprehensive pictures of the kidneys by combining X-rays and computer technologies. This test may assist examine the size and shape of the kidneys, as well as identify renal disease such as the existence of tumors, cysts, or kidney stones. Kidney impairment can be caused by a number of factors, including diabetes, high blood pressure, and obesity.

- Magnetic Resonance Imaging (MRI): An MRI creates comprehensive pictures of the kidneys by using a magnetic field and radio waves. This test may assist analyze the size and form of the kidneys, as well as identify renal abnormalities such as the presence of tumors, cysts, or kidney stones. Kidney damage can be detected with this test.

- Renal Scan: A renal scan is a nuclear medicine test that produces pictures of the kidneys by making use of a tiny quantity of radioactive material. This test is known as a renal scintigraphy. This test may assist in the diagnosis of kidney disease, including but not limited to a reduction in blood flow to the kidneys or obstructions in the urinary system.

Imaging examinations like these may assist in the diagnosis of kidney disease as well as the monitoring of its development. In the event that you are having any symptoms or have any risk factors for kidney disease, it is imperative that you consult with your healthcare professional to decide whether or not imaging tests are required.

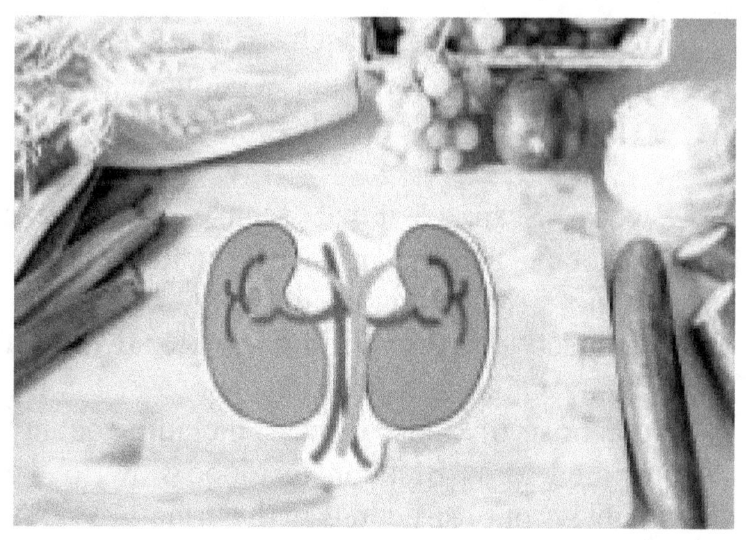

Chapter 4: Traditional Treatment Options for Kidney Disease

Medications to manage kidney disease

Medications of many kinds may be used in the treatment and management of renal disease. The precise medication(s) that are advised will be determined by the root cause of the kidney illness as well as the stage of the condition. Medications such as the following are among the most often prescribed treatments for renal disease:

- These drugs, known as ACE inhibitors and ARBs, are often prescribed to patients who suffer from renal disease in order to bring their blood pressure under control. They are effective because they relax the blood arteries and lessen the workload placed on the heart to circulate blood throughout the body. The quantity of protein that is lost in the urine may be reduced by using ACE inhibitors or ARBs, which can also help protect the kidneys from damage.

- Diuretics are drugs that assist the body in excreting excess fluid and salt, and their common name is "water pills." They are often used in the treatment of cardiovascular conditions like as heart failure and high blood pressure, both of which are major consequences of renal disease.

- Erythropoietin-stimulating agents, sometimes known as ESAs, are as follows: ESAs are drugs that promote the synthesis of red blood cells and are known as erythropoiesis-stimulating agents. They are often used as a treatment for anemia in patients who suffer from renal illness.

- Phosphate binders are drugs that assist manage the amount of phosphorus that is present in the blood. Phosphate binders are also known as phosphate chelators. They do this by attaching themselves to phosphorus in the digestive tract, so blocking the element's absorption into the circulation. Those who already have renal illness are at risk for developing bone disease because they have high blood levels of the mineral phosphorus.

- Statins are a kind of drug that helps reduce the levels of cholesterol that are found in the blood. They are often used in the treatment of excessive cholesterol levels in patients with renal disease, which may assist in lowering the risk of cardiovascular disease.

It is essential to have a solid working relationship with a healthcare professional in order to decide which medications will be most effective in the management of renal disease. When the condition continues to worsen over time, it is possible that the medications may need to be modified.

Dialysis

Dialysis is a therapy that is performed when the kidneys are no longer able to fulfill the job of filtering waste materials and excess fluids from the circulation. This occurs when kidney disease develops. Dialysis may be broken down into its two primary subtypes: hemodialysis and peritoneal dialysis.

Hemodialysis:
During the process of hemodialysis, blood is drawn from the patient and routed via a device known as a dialyzer, which functions in the same way that an artificial kidney would. The blood is sent through a

dialyzer, which removes toxins and extra fluids from the blood before sending it back into the body.

Hemodialysis is commonly performed three times each week for anything between three and five hours per session. The individual's degree of renal function as well as their general state of health will determine the frequency of dialysis treatments as well as their length.

Peritoneal dialysis:
Peritoneal dialysis involves inserting a catheter into the abdomen, after which a specialized fluid is administered into the peritoneal cavity via the catheter. The fluid remains in the abdominal cavity for a few hours, during which time it is able to soak up waste materials and excess fluid that have been drawn from the blood. After this, the fluid is drained from the abdomen, and it is then replaced with new fluid. Since it may be performed at home and on a daily basis, peritoneal dialysis enables patients to get treatment more often than hemodialysis does.

When can you finally discontinue the dialysis treatment? If the patient's kidneys begin to operate normally again, it is feasible that they will no longer need dialysis treatment. This process is referred to as renal recovery. On the other hand, this circumstance is very unusual and almost never happens until the underlying cause of the renal illness is effectively cured. Dialysis is a therapy that will often need to be continued for the rest of a person's life if they have end-stage renal disease.

Those who have renal disease that has progressed to its last stage may, in certain instances, be candidates for a kidney transplant. In a kidney transplant, the diseased kidney is removed and replaced with a healthy kidney obtained from a donor. On the other hand, not everyone is eligible for a kidney transplant, and there may be a significant amount of time spent on the waiting list before one can be performed.

Dialysis is a therapy that is used to eliminate waste products and excess fluids from the blood when the kidneys are unable to accomplish this job on their own. In a nutshell, dialysis is a treatment. The two most common forms of dialysis are hemodialysis and peritoneal dialysis. The frequency and length of dialysis treatment will vary from patient to patient based on their degree of kidney function as well as their general state of health. Those who have renal disease that has progressed to its last stage often need to undergo dialysis for the rest of their lives.

Kidney transplant

Those who have reached the end stage of renal disease may be candidates for a kidney transplant, which is a surgical operation in which a healthy kidney obtained from a donor is implanted into a recipient who has advanced kidney disease. The newly transplanted kidney takes over the function of the recipient's failing kidneys, allowing them to avoid the need for dialysis treatment.

When a person reaches the end stage of renal disease, which is defined as when the kidneys perform at less than 10-15% of their normal capacity, kidney transplantation becomes a viable treatment option. Those who have specific kidney illnesses, such as polycystic kidney disease, that may reoccur after a transplant may potentially be candidates for kidney transplantation as an additional treatment option.

The kidney transplant operation typically lasts between three and four hours and is performed under general anesthesia. The replacement kidney will be positioned in the patient's lower abdomen, and the surgeon will link it to the patient's blood vessels as well as the urinary system. Unless they are creating complications for the patient, such as high blood pressure or infections, the patient's own kidneys are often kept in situ.

After the surgical procedure, the individual will be required to take medicine in order to prevent their body from rejecting the new kidney. Some drugs have the potential to depress the immune system, which may result in adverse consequences such as an increased risk of infections and cancer. For the purpose of ensuring that the replacement kidney is operating appropriately and for the purpose of adjusting the dose of any drugs, routine monitoring and blood tests are required.

The success of a kidney transplant is determined by a number of variables, including the age and general health of the recipient, the condition of the kidney that is given, and the degree to which the donor and recipient are compatible with one another. The longevity of a transplanted kidney ranges anywhere from ten to fifteen years, with some kidneys having a substantially longer lifespan than others. If the kidney that was donated does not function well, the recipient may have to restart their dialysis treatment or they may be eligible for a second transplant.

It is reasonable to anticipate that the recipient will see a significant improvement in their overall health after a kidney transplant that is successful. They will no longer need dialysis and will be able to return to their usual lifestyle, but they will have to take drugs for the rest of their lives to prevent their body from rejecting the new kidney.

Chapter 5: Lifestyle Changes to Reverse Kidney Disease

Alterations to one's way of life, in conjunction with medical therapy, have the potential to play a significant part in the reversal of renal disease. Alterations to one's diet, regular exercise program, and behaviors such as smoking and drinking alcohol intake might be among these alterations. Making these adjustments may help to alleviate the strain that is being placed on the kidneys, improve overall health, and control symptoms. In the chapters that follow, we will discuss the modifications to one's way of life that may be implemented to stop the progression of renal disease.

Diet modifications for kidney health

Food is an essential component in the treatment of renal disease as well as its potential reversal. Although there are certain meals and drinks that may exacerbate the status of the kidneys and put more burden on them, there are other foods and beverages that can assist decrease inflammation and enhance renal function. In this chapter, we will discuss the dietary adjustments that may be performed to reverse renal disease and enhance kidney health.

Reducing Sodium Intake

Reducing the amount of salt consumed is one of the most important dietary adjustments that can be done to enhance kidney function. Since sodium may cause the body to retain extra fluids, it can place additional stress on the kidneys, which can make the disease even worse. Those who have renal illness should try to limit their daily salt intake to no more than 2,000 mg as much as possible. This may be accomplished by avoiding foods that have been processed, foods stored in cans, and foods that have a high salt content. Instead, individuals should choose for fresh fruits and vegetables, leaner cuts of meat, and alternatives with less salt.

Decreasing one's consumption of protein

Reducing the amount of protein consumed is another dietary adjustment that may be performed to promote kidney function. Protein is necessary for the growth and maintenance of tissues, however consuming an excessive amount might place extra stress on the kidneys. Individuals who have renal illness should try to limit the amount of protein they eat each day to no more than 0.8 grams per kilogram of body weight. This may be accomplished by consuming a lower quantity of proteins derived from animals, such as meat, eggs, and dairy, while simultaneously consuming a higher quantity of proteins derived from plants, such as beans, lentils, and tofu.

Increasing One's Consumption of Fiber
Raising the amount of fiber you consume each day may also assist enhance kidney health. Fiber helps to decrease inflammation and may assist in the regulation of blood sugar levels, both of which may help to lower the amount of stress placed on the kidneys. Those who suffer from renal illness should make it a point to eat between 20 and 30 grams of fiber on a daily basis. This goal may be met by increasing the number of whole grains, fruits, and vegetables consumed.

lowering one's consumption of phosphorus.
Another major dietary modification that can be done to promote kidney function is to reduce the amount of phosphorus that is consumed on a daily basis. A diet that contains an excessive amount of phosphorus may cause the body to excrete calcium, which can lead to brittle bones and make renal disease worse. Individuals who have renal illness should try to limit their daily phosphorus intake to between 800 and 1,000 mg as much as possible.

This may be accomplished by avoiding processed meals, soft drinks, and foods that are rich in phosphorus including dairy products, meat, and poultry. Moreover, it is important to stay away from foods that have added sugar.

An Increase in the Use of Antioxidants
Raising the amount of antioxidants, you take in on a regular basis may also aid boost kidney health. Antioxidants aid to minimize inflammation and defend against the damaging effects of oxidative stress, both of which may be caused by free radicals. Those who suffer from kidney illness should make it a priority to eat foods that are rich in antioxidants. Some examples of these foods are beans, berries, and dark leafy greens.

Hydration
In addition, enough water is essential for healthy kidney function. Consuming a lot of water might aid in the flushing out of toxins and lower the likelihood of developing kidney stones. Those who suffer from renal illness should make it a point to consume at least 8 to 10 glasses of water each day, and even more if they have diarrhea or are perspiring heavily.

Alchohol consumption
Consuming alcohol in moderation is also essential for maintaining healthy kidneys. Consuming an

excessive amount of alcohol may cause harm to the kidneys and make renal disease worse. Women with renal illness should restrict their alcohol intake to no more than one drink per day, while males with kidney disease should limit themselves to no more than two drinks per day.

Conclusion

To summarize, making adjustments to one's diet may be an efficient and fruitful strategy to enhance kidney health and even reverse renal disease. Important dietary changes that can be made to improve kidney health include reducing the amount of sodium and protein consumed, increasing the amount of fiber consumed, reducing the amount of phosphorus consumed, increasing the amount of antioxidants consumed, remaining hydrated, and limiting the amount of alcohol consumed. Individuals who suffer from renal disease should see both their primary care physician and a certified dietitian in order to build a bespoke eating strategy that caters to their individual requirements and objectives.

Exercise and physical activity

Exercise and physical activity are crucial for maintaining overall health and well-being, and this is especially true for individuals with kidney disease. Regular exercise has been shown to provide numerous benefits for individuals with kidney disease, including improved cardiovascular health, better blood sugar control, and even a slower progression of kidney disease. In this section, we will explore how exercise and physical activity can help in reversing kidney diseases.

Benefits of Exercise for Kidney Health:
- Improved Cardiovascular Health: Kidney disease is often associated with an increased risk of heart disease. Exercise can help improve cardiovascular health by lowering blood pressure, improving blood sugar control, and reducing inflammation. Regular exercise can also help reduce the risk of heart disease by improving lipid profiles, decreasing triglycerides, and increasing HDL (good cholesterol) levels.
- Better Blood Sugar Control: High blood sugar levels can damage blood vessels and

lead to kidney damage. Regular exercise can help improve blood sugar control by increasing insulin sensitivity, which allows the body to better regulate blood sugar levels.

- Slower Progression of Kidney Disease: Regular exercise has been shown to slow the progression of kidney disease in some individuals. One study found that individuals who engaged in regular exercise had a 20-30% lower risk of developing end-stage kidney disease compared to those who were sedentary.

- Improved Mental Health: Exercise can help improve mental health by reducing stress, anxiety, and depression. Individuals with kidney disease may experience emotional distress due to the impact of the disease on their daily lives. Engaging in regular exercise can help alleviate these symptoms and improve overall quality of life.

Types of Exercise for Kidney Health:

- Aerobic Exercise: Aerobic exercise, such as walking, running, cycling, or swimming, is an excellent way to improve cardiovascular health and overall fitness. It is recommended that individuals engage in at least 150 minutes of moderate-intensity aerobic exercise per week.

- Resistance Training: Resistance training, such as weightlifting, can help improve muscle strength and mass. It is recommended that individuals engage in resistance training at least twice per week.
- Flexibility Training: Flexibility training, such as stretching or yoga, can help improve flexibility and mobility. It is recommended that individuals engage in flexibility training at least two to three times per week.

Precautions for Exercise and Kidney Disease:
Individuals with kidney disease should always consult with their healthcare provider before starting an exercise program.

There are some precautions that individuals with kidney disease should take when engaging in exercise:

- Avoid high-impact activities: High-impact activities, such as jumping or running, can be hard on the joints and may cause injury.
- Avoid dehydration: Individuals with kidney disease are at increased risk of dehydration.

It is important to drink plenty of fluids before, during, and after exercise.

- Avoid overexertion: Individuals with kidney disease may experience fatigue more easily. It is important to listen to your body and avoid overexertion.

- Avoid activities that may cause injury: Individuals with kidney disease may have an increased risk of bone fractures. It is important to avoid activities that may cause injury, such as contact sports or high-intensity activities.

In conclusion, exercise and physical activity are essential components of a healthy lifestyle, and they are especially important for individuals with kidney disease. Regular exercise has been shown to provide numerous benefits, including improved cardiovascular health, better blood sugar control, and even a slower progression of kidney disease. Individuals with kidney disease should always consult with their healthcare provider before starting an exercise program and should take precautions to avoid injury and dehydration. With proper guidance and precautions, exercise can be a safe and effective way to improve kidney health and reverse kidney diseases.

Managing high blood pressure and diabetes

Diabetes and high blood pressure are two of the most common factors that contribute to renal damage. Thus, proper management of these disorders is very necessary for avoiding and treating renal disease. Managing high blood pressure and diabetes in order to protect kidney health may be done in a few different ways:

<u>Controlling High Blood Pressure</u>

- Having high blood pressure, also known as hypertension, may be harmful to the kidneys because it decreases the amount of blood that flows to them. This forces the kidneys to work harder and less effectively, which can lead to kidney damage. The following are some methods that may be used to control high blood pressure:

- Always follow your doctor's instructions while taking prescribed medicine. Using antihypertensive medication as directed may assist in the regulation of blood pressure and lower the risk of kidney damage. It is quite necessary to take these drugs exactly as directed by the physician.

- Adopting a diet that is low in salt, fat, and cholesterol is one of the best things you can do to help decrease your blood pressure. Fruits and vegetables, as well as other foods that are high in potassium content, are another potential source of assistance.

- Frequent exercise may help decrease blood pressure by increasing the strength and function of the heart and blood arteries. If you exercise regularly, you can help lower your blood pressure.

- Take steps to manage your stress: extended periods of stress have been linked to increased blood pressure. The management of stress may be assisted by practices such as yoga, meditation, and deep breathing.

Managing diabetes:
Diabetes may cause damage to the blood vessels and nerves that govern kidney function, which can lead to kidney damage. Controlling diabetes is important to prevent kidney damage.

The following are some methods that may be used to control diabetes:

- Always follow your doctor's instructions while taking prescribed medications. Medicines such as insulin and oral hypoglycemic agents may assist in controlling blood sugar levels and preventing kidney damage if they are used as directed. It is quite necessary to take these drugs exactly as directed by the physician.

- Adopt a Healthy Food Adopting a diet that is rich in fiber and low in carbs will help regulate blood sugar levels. Meals that are high in protein and low in fat, such as fish, tofu, and lean cuts of meat, may also be beneficial.

- Regular exercise may help regulate blood sugar levels by enhancing insulin sensitivity and increasing glucose uptake. This can be accomplished by regular exercise.

- Keep an Eye on Your Blood Sugar Levels Keeping an eye on your blood sugar levels and monitoring them on a regular basis will help you recognize and better control changes in your blood sugar levels.

- Take Care of Your Weight: Keeping your weight at a healthy level will assist in the regulation of blood sugar levels as well as the reduction of the risk of kidney damage.

In conclusion, it is essential to treat both high blood pressure and diabetes in order to avoid kidney damage and to reverse its effects. Controlling these problems and maintaining good kidney health may be accomplished with the use of medicine, adopting healthy behaviors, and undergoing routine monitoring.

Quitting smoking

Smoking is a well-known risk factor for a wide range of health problems, including kidney disease. Smoking can harm the kidneys in several ways, and quitting smoking can be an essential step in reversing kidney disease.

- How Does Smoking Harm the Kidneys? Smoking can damage the kidneys in several ways, including:

- Reduced Blood Flow: Smoking causes the blood vessels to narrow, reducing blood flow to the kidneys. This reduction in blood flow can cause the kidneys to work less efficiently and can lead to kidney damage.
- Increased Blood Pressure: Smoking can cause an increase in blood pressure, which can damage the blood vessels in the kidneys and lead to kidney damage.
- Increased Risk of Kidney Disease: Smoking increases the risk of developing kidney disease, particularly in people with other risk factors such as diabetes and high blood pressure.

Accelerated Decline in Kidney Function: Smoking can accelerate the decline in kidney function, particularly in people with pre-existing kidney disease.

How Does Quitting Smoking Help Reverse Kidney Disease?

Quitting smoking can be an essential step in reversing kidney disease, as it can help to:

- Improve Blood Flow: Quitting smoking can help to improve blood flow to the kidneys, which can help to improve kidney function.
- Reduce Blood Pressure: Quitting smoking can help to reduce blood pressure, which can help to protect the blood vessels in the kidneys and prevent kidney damage.
- Slow the Progression of Kidney Disease: Quitting smoking can help to slow the progression of kidney disease, particularly in people with pre-existing kidney disease.
- Reduce the Risk of Kidney Failure: Quitting smoking can help to reduce the risk of kidney failure, which can be a serious and life-threatening complication of kidney disease.
- Improve Overall Health: Quitting smoking can help to improve overall health, which can help to reduce the risk of developing other health problems that can affect kidney function, such as diabetes and high blood pressure.

How to Quit Smoking?

Quitting smoking can be challenging, but there are many resources available to help. Some strategies for quitting smoking include:

- Nicotine Replacement Therapy: Nicotine Replacement Therapy (NRT) is a commonly used method to help individuals quit smoking. It works by delivering nicotine to the body through gum, patches, or other methods, which can reduce withdrawal symptoms and make it easier to quit smoking. NRT is available over the counter, and it is generally safe and effective when used as directed. However, it is important to consult with a healthcare provider before using NRT, especially if you have underlying medical conditions.

- Prescription medications: Prescription medications such as bupropion and varenicline can also be effective in helping individuals quit smoking. Bupropion works by reducing cravings and withdrawal symptoms, while varenicline works by blocking the effects of nicotine on the brain. These medications should be prescribed and closely monitored by a healthcare provider, as they may have side effects and can interact with other medications.

- Behavioral therapy: Behavioral therapy can also be an effective tool for quitting smoking. Cognitive-behavioral therapy, for example, can help individuals identify triggers that may lead to smoking and develop coping strategies to deal with cravings and stress. This type of therapy can be conducted in individual or group sessions and is typically provided by a mental health professional.

- Support groups can also provide a valuable source of support and encouragement for individuals trying to quit smoking. Nicotine Anonymous, for example, is a 12-step program similar to Alcoholics Anonymous that focuses on helping individuals quit smoking and maintain their abstinence. Support groups can provide a safe and supportive environment for individuals to share their experiences, receive guidance and advice, and connect with others who are going through similar struggles.

- Finally, making lifestyle changes such as getting regular exercise, eating a healthy diet, and managing stress can also help to reduce cravings and make it easier to quit smoking. Exercise can help to reduce stress and anxiety, which can be triggers for smoking, while a healthy diet can provide the nutrients and energy needed to support a successful quit attempt. Stress management techniques such as meditation, deep breathing, or yoga can also be helpful in reducing stress and promoting relaxation.

In summary, quitting smoking is a complex and challenging process, and there are many different methods and strategies that can be used to increase the chances of success. Nicotine replacement therapy, prescription medications, behavioral therapy, support groups, and lifestyle changes can all be effective tools in helping individuals quit smoking and reverse the harmful effects of smoking on the kidneys and overall health. It is important to work closely with a healthcare provider and to develop a comprehensive plan that addresses the unique needs and circumstances of each individual.

Reducing alcohol intake

Consuming alcohol is a prevalent practice in many countries around the globe; yet, doing so regularly might have negative consequences on kidney health. Consuming an excessive amount of alcohol may result in damage to the kidneys, including acute renal injury and chronic kidney disease. The kidneys are responsible for removing waste products and toxins from the blood, and they play an important part in this process.

Dehydration, which alcohol may induce, can lead to a reduction in blood flow to the kidneys, which can damage the kidneys' capacity to function correctly. Alcohol can also produce nausea and vomiting. In addition, drinking alcohol may induce changes in the structure and function of the kidneys, such as inflammation, scarring, and oxidative stress, all of which can, over the course of time, result in chronic renal disease.

A significant reduction in alcohol use is one of the most important steps that can be taken to both stop and reverse kidney damage. Alcohol intake should be limited to no more than one drink per day for women and no more than two drinks per day for men, according to the recommendations. Nonetheless, even low to moderate alcohol use may be detrimental for persons who have renal disease, and it is suggested that these individuals entirely refrain from alcohol consumption.

Reducing the amount of alcohol consumed may help reverse renal disease in a number of different ways, including the following:

- Reducing dehydration: As was noted previously, alcohol may induce dehydration, which can affect kidney function. Nevertheless, dehydration can be prevented by drinking less water. You can assist maintain appropriate amounts of hydration and promote good kidney function by lowering the amount of alcohol that you consume.

- Blood pressure reduction: Drinking an excessive amount of alcohol may cause blood pressure to rise, which can result in kidney damage if left untreated. You may assist in lowering your blood pressure and preventing future damage to the kidneys by minimizing the amount of alcohol that you consume.

- Lowering oxidative stress is important since drinking alcohol may lead to an increase in oxidative stress, which can be harmful to the cells and tissues throughout the body, including the kidneys. You may aid in the reduction of oxidative stress and maintain healthy kidney function by cutting down on your use of alcohol.

- Prevention of liver disease: Drinking too much alcohol may induce liver disease, which in turn can cause damage to the kidneys. You can assist avoid liver disease and protect the kidneys from additional damage if you cut down on the amount of alcohol you consume.

Alterations to one's diet and other aspects of one's lifestyle, in addition to lowering one's alcohol use, may also aid improve one's kidney health. Among them include keeping a healthy weight, being physically active on a regular basis, and eating a diet that is both balanced and nutritious. If you have been given a diagnosis of kidney disease, it is essential to work closely with your healthcare practitioner to build a specific treatment plan. This treatment plan should include adjustments to your food and lifestyle, as well as medication if it is deemed appropriate.

In a nutshell, cutting down on one's use of alcoholic beverages is one of the most important things that can be done to both stop and reverse kidney damage. You can help maintain correct hydration levels, decrease blood pressure, reduce oxidative stress, and avoid liver disease by lowering the amount of alcohol you consume, all of which may help support healthy kidney function. If you are having trouble cutting down on the amount of alcohol you consume, it may be good to seek professional assistance, such as counseling or support groups, to assist you on your road toward better kidney health.

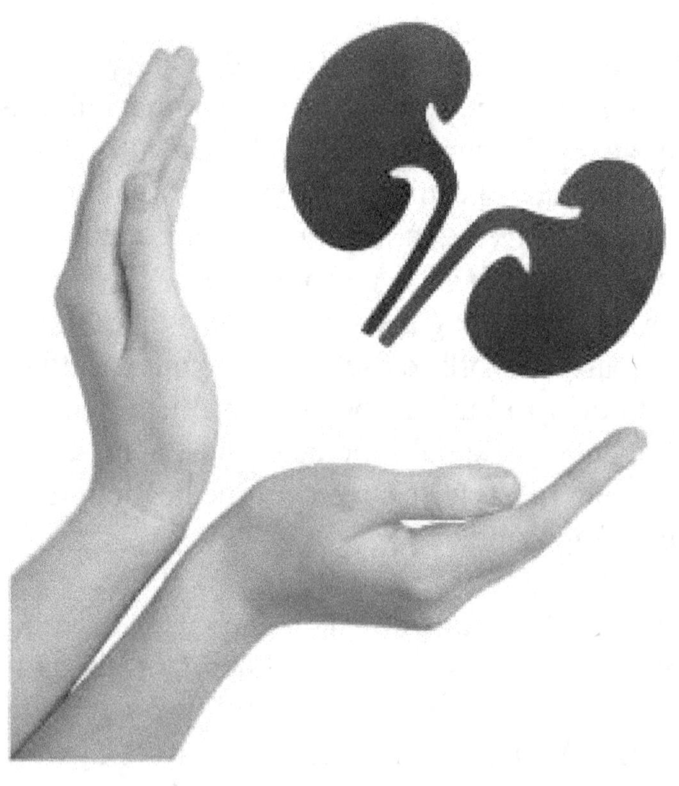

Chapter 6: Alternative and Complementary Therapies for Kidney Disease

Herbal supplements and traditional medicine

An increasing number of people are turning to alternative treatments, such as herbal supplements and traditional medicine, in order to treat renal illness. Some of these treatments have been around for centuries, while others are very new and have not been subjected to much research since they were first introduced. In the following paragraphs, we are going to talk about the use of herbal supplements and traditional medicine for renal illness, including the possible advantages and dangers associated with these treatments.

<u>Herbal Supplements for Conditions Affecting the Kidneys:</u>

- Astragalus: Astragalus is a well-known plant that plays an important role in traditional Chinese medicine, serving to both strengthen the immune system and enhance kidney function. It is thought to act by boosting the generation of white blood cells, which are essential to the immune system's ability to combat infections. Astragalus has been proven to enhance kidney function in patients with chronic kidney disease (CKD) by lowering levels of inflammation and oxidative stress, according to the findings of a few research.

- Ginger: Ginger is a spice that is used often and it contains qualities that may reduce inflammation. In animal research, it has been shown to decrease inflammation and oxidative stress, and in some limited human trials, it has been demonstrated that it can enhance kidney function in persons who have CKD. On the other hand, there is a need for more study to assess the long-term effects of ginger on the health of the kidneys.

- Turmeric: Indian cuisine makes extensive use of turmeric as a seasoning ingredient. It is rich in curcumin, a substance with anti-inflammatory and antioxidant effects, which is found in turmeric. Curcumin has been found in a few trials to enhance kidney function in patients with chronic kidney disease (CKD) by lowering inflammatory and oxidative stress levels.

- Milk Thistle: Milk thistle is a medicinal herb that has been used for the treatment of liver and kidney conditions for hundreds of years. It is rich in silymarin, a chemical with anti-inflammatory and antioxidant effects that may be found in the plant. Milk thistle has been demonstrated in a number of trials to enhance kidney function in persons who have chronic kidney disease (CKD) by lowering inflammatory and oxidative stress levels.

- Cordyceps: Cordyceps is a kind of fungus that has been used in traditional Chinese medicine to treat a wide range of conditions, including kidney failure. Polysaccharides and other substances found in it have anti-inflammatory and antioxidant capabilities, and they are present in the substance. Cordyceps have been demonstrated to enhance renal function in CKD patients by lowering inflammatory markers and oxidative stress, according to the findings of a few studies.

- Dandelion: The diuretic qualities of dandelion are thought to aid kidney function by stimulating the production of urine and hastening their clearance from the body. Moreover, dandelion is an excellent source of antioxidants, which, when consumed, may assist in the prevention of oxidative damage to the kidneys.

- Nettle: The plant nettle has a long history of usage in many forms of traditional medicine for the treatment of a variety of diseases and ailments, including kidney dysfunction. Nettle is thought to contain qualities that make it a diuretic, and these features may help decrease inflammation in the kidneys, enhance kidney function, and lower proteinuria in people who suffer from kidney disease.

- Saw palmetto: Saw palmetto is a herb that is often used in the treatment of prostate enlargement; however, there is some evidence to suggest that it may also be beneficial to kidney function. It is thought that saw palmetto has anti-inflammatory qualities, which may help to decrease inflammation in the kidneys and enhance renal function. Saw palmetto may be found at health food stores.

<u>Alternative and Traditional Treatment for Kidney Conditions:</u>

- Traditional Chinese Medicine: The term "Traditional Chinese Medicine" (often abbreviated as "TCM") refers to a holistic medical practice that has been practiced in China for thousands of years. Acupuncture, herbal medicine, and food therapy are all components of this treatment. TCM practitioners believe that kidney illness is caused by imbalances in the body, and as a result, they use a mix of acupuncture, herbal medicine, and nutritional treatment in order to enhance kidney function and restore balance.

- Ayurveda: The Indian subcontinent is the birthplace of the age-old medical practice known as ayurveda. Herbal medication, nutritional treatment, and behavioral adjustments are all components of this approach. Ayurveda practitioners believe that kidney illness is caused by imbalances in the body. Because of this belief, they use a mix of herbal medication, nutritional treatment, and lifestyle adjustments in order to restore balance and enhance kidney function.

Risks of Traditional Medicine and Herbal Supplements

Although while many herbal supplements and traditional treatments are thought to be risk-free, there is always the possibility that they might cause undesirable reactions or side effects. Certain herbs have the potential to interact negatively with other drugs, while others may provoke allergic responses or toxicity in the body. There is a possibility of contamination and adulteration while using traditional medicines like TCM and Ayurveda since these types of treatments are not subject to the same rigorous standards of regulation as Western medicine.

It is essential to see a medical professional before beginning treatment with any herbal supplements or traditional remedies, and this is particularly the case if you have renal disease or are already on medication. Your healthcare practitioner should be able to assist you in identifying any possible hazards and verify that any remedies you use do not interact negatively with any drugs or other treatments you are already receiving.

Acupuncture

Acupuncture is a traditional Chinese medical practice that includes inserting tiny needles into certain body sites. It is thought that acupuncture works by triggering the body's natural healing mechanisms and enhancing the circulation of energy, also known as "qi," throughout the body.

Acupuncture has been shown to reduce symptoms of renal illness and enhance kidney function by lowering inflammation, increasing blood flow, and modulating the immune system. Acupuncture may also be helpful in reducing the symptoms of renal disease treatments, such as tiredness and nausea, which may be a burden for patients.

There have been a number of investigations on the possible therapeutic effects of acupuncture for renal illness. For instance, a study that was conducted in 2014 and published in the Journal of Traditional Chinese Medicine discovered that the combination of acupuncture and medication was more effective than medication alone at improving kidney function and reducing proteinuria (excess protein in the urine) in patients who suffered from chronic kidney disease.

Another study that was conducted and published in the year 2017 in the Journal of Acupuncture and Meridian Studies found that acupuncture may help to alleviate symptoms of kidney disease, such as fatigue, by regulating the function of the adrenal glands, which are involved in the stress response of the body.

Even though there hasn't been a lot of study done on acupuncture as a treatment for kidney illness yet, it seems like it might be a useful supplemental therapy for individuals who have the condition. Nonetheless, patients should always speak with their healthcare professional before beginning acupuncture therapy, just as they should do before beginning treatment with herbal supplements or conventional medication.

Massage therapy

To enhance blood flow, relieve muscular tension, and promote relaxation, one kind of manual treatment known as massage therapy includes the manipulation of the soft tissues of the body. Those who suffer from renal disease may reap some health benefits by participating in a variety of massage modalities, including the following:

Swedish massage: This is the most popular kind of massage, and it includes kneading, circular motions, and long, flowing strokes that are performed on the surface layers of the muscles. Relaxation, less tension, and improved circulation are among potential benefits of doing so.

Deep tissue massage: In order to reach the deepest levels of muscle and connective tissue, this particular kind of massage employs slow strokes and deep finger pressure. It may assist in relieving chronic muscular tension, enhancing flexibility, and lowering inflammation.

Reflexology: This kind of massage method includes applying pressure to certain areas on the feet, hands, or ears that correlate to various sections of the body, one of which being the kidneys. Both your circulation and your stress levels may improve as a result.

While treating kidney illness with massage therapy, the therapist may concentrate on massaging certain parts of the body in order to improve kidney function and lessen the severity of the symptoms. They may, for instance, massage the lower back, which is the region in which the kidneys are found, or the feet, which have numerous acupressure sites that are considered to be associated to kidney health. Another option is to massage the abdomen, which is the area in which the kidneys are placed.

It is essential to stress that massage therapy is not intended to serve as a replacement for conventional medical treatment in the case of renal illness. Those who have renal illness should talk to their primary care physician before beginning any new alternative treatment, including massage. This is the recommended course of action. Also, persons who have specific medical disorders, such as blood clots or infections, may not be good candidates for massage therapy. Because of this, it is essential to clarify any concerns with the therapist before beginning the massage therapy session.

Yoga and meditation

The practices of yoga and meditation have been found to have a number of health advantages, including the reduction of stress, the improvement of mood, and the enhancement of physical fitness. Perhaps, these benefits might also apply to people with renal illness.

The physical postures, breathing exercises, and meditation or relaxation techniques that make up yoga are all components of the mind-body practice known as yoga. It has been shown to assist in lowering levels of stress and anxiety, enhancing physical function, and bringing down levels of inflammation in the body. Due to the fact that stress and inflammation may contribute to the advancement of kidney disease, people who already have the condition may find these advantages to be especially beneficial.

Some yoga poses that may be beneficial for patients with kidney disease include:

- Child's pose (Balasana): This pose can help to stretch the hips, thighs, and ankles while promoting relaxation and reducing stress.
- Cat-Cow pose (Marjaryasana-Bitilasana): This pose can help to improve spinal mobility and circulation, while also promoting relaxation and stress reduction.
- Warrior II pose (Virabhadrasana II): This pose can help to strengthen the legs and improve balance, while also promoting relaxation and reducing stress.

Meditation is a practice that entails training the mind to concentrate on the present moment, generally via the use of breathing exercises or mental images. This training is done in order to benefit from the benefits of meditation. It has been shown to aid in the alleviation of stress and anxiety, the promotion of better sleep, and an overall improvement in well-being. Those afflicted with kidney illness may benefit greatly from the practice of meditation, since stress and worry have been shown to speed up the course of the condition.

One of the most frequent kinds of meditation is called mindfulness meditation, and it requires the meditator to focus on the here and now while suspending all judgment. This may help to alleviate feelings of tension and worry, lift mood, and enhance sensations of relaxation and overall well-being. One may engage in the practice of mindfulness meditation in a number of different environments, including one's own home, in a classroom setting with other people, or by listening to guided meditations that are accessible online.

Overall, adding yoga and meditation into a treatment plan for renal illness may bring a variety of potential advantages to both the patient's physical and mental health. Individuals should always check with their healthcare professional before starting a new exercise or meditation practice, particularly if they have any underlying health disorders or concerns. This is especially important for patients who have a history of cardiovascular disease.

Chapter 7: Managing Stress and Mental Health

How stress affects kidney disease

The presence of stress in one's life is inescapable, and it has the potential to adversely affect both one's physical and mental health. When stress is allowed to persist for an extended period of time or becomes chronic, it may bring about a broad variety of unfavorable results for one's health, including the onset and progression of kidney disease. In this piece, we will go further into the ways in which stress manifests itself physically in the kidneys.

It is vital to have a solid understanding of the physiological processes at play in order to have a solid understanding of how stress affects the kidneys. The body reacts to stress by stimulating the sympathetic nervous system and releasing stress hormones like cortisol and adrenaline into the bloodstream. This is known as the "fight or flight" reaction. These hormones cause a cascade of physiological changes in the body, including an increase in the pace at which the person breathes, their heart rate, and their blood pressure.

These alterations have the potential to become permanent when the body is subjected to prolonged stress, which may cause long-term harm to a variety of organs, including the kidneys. Alterations in the blood flow to the kidneys, which may be brought on by persistent stress, can bring to a slowing down of the kidneys' filtration rate. This slowing down of the filtration rate may cause a buildup of waste materials in the blood, which can ultimately result in the development of renal disease.

In addition, persistent stress may produce inflammation in the kidneys, which can result in damage to the renal tissues and a reduction in the kidneys' capacity to perform their functions normally. Chronic inflammation may also lead to the generation of free radicals, which can cause oxidative damage to the kidneys and speed up the course of renal disease. Free radicals can be produced when there is an increase in white blood cell count.

The development of high blood pressure, which is one of the most important risk factors for kidney disease, has been linked to stress as another potential contributor. Chronic stress can cause the release of hormones that increase blood pressure, which can damage the blood vessels in the kidneys and impair their ability to filter waste products out of the blood. This damage can be caused by the kidneys' inability to properly filter out the harmful substances in the blood.

In addition, stress may influence behaviors and lifestyle variables, both of which are known to have a role in the progression of renal disease. For instance, stress may lead to bad eating habits, such as consuming excessive quantities of salt and sugar, which can contribute to the development of high blood pressure and renal disease. Stress can also lead to a decrease in the immune system's ability to fight against infections. It is also possible for stress to have a role in the development of unhealthy coping methods, such as the habit of smoking or drinking excessive amounts of alcohol, both of which may further harm the kidneys.

In general, prolonged exposure to stress may have a major influence on the kidneys, which can ultimately contribute to the onset and progression of renal disease. Those who suffer from renal illness should make it a priority to reduce their levels of stress via the practice of a variety of relaxation methods, such as yoga, meditation, or massage treatment. Individuals have the ability to enhance their general health and lower the risk of problems connected with renal disease by taking steps to manage their levels of stress.

Techniques to manage stress and anxiety

Both our physical and emotional health may be negatively impacted by worry and stress, and this includes the kidneys' ability to function normally. The good news is that there are a variety of strategies that can be used for the management of stress and anxiety, which, in turn, may assist in the improvement of kidney health. We will talk about some of the most effective methods.

<u>Mindfulness meditation:</u>
The practice of mindfulness meditation is directing your attention to the here and now while embracing your thoughts and emotions in an open and non-judgmental manner. This may assist in lowering levels of tension and anxiety by increasing feelings of relaxation and decreasing the inclination to dwell on unfavorable thoughts and feelings. Choose a spot that is calm and comfortable for you to sit or lay down in so that you may practice mindfulness meditation there. Next, direct your attention to your breath or a mantra. Whenever you find that your mind has wandered, just bring it back to the breath or mantra that you are focusing on.

<u>Yoga:</u>
Breathing exercises, meditation, and various physical postures are all components of the practice

of yoga, which has both a physical and a spiritual component. The practice of yoga may assist in alleviating stress and anxiety by facilitating relaxation, enhancing circulation, and lowering levels of muscular tension, among other benefits. In addition, yoga may be adapted to fulfill the requirements of those who suffer from renal illness by excluding the postures that are likely to place an excessive amount of pressure on the organs. Before beginning a yoga practice, it is highly important to first have a conversation with a trained yoga teacher who has prior experience dealing with patients diagnosed with renal illness.

Progressive muscular relaxation:
In order to facilitate relaxation and lessen the amount of muscular tension, a technique known as progressive muscle relaxation involves tensing and then releasing particular muscle groups. With the promotion of relaxation and the reduction of muscular tension, this method may be useful in the reduction of stress and anxiety. Choose a calm and comfortable area to sit or lay down in order to practice progressive muscle relaxation. Next, concentrate your attention on each individual muscle group, first tensing the muscles for a few seconds and then releasing that tension.

Deep breathing:
The practice of taking lengthy, slow breaths, sometimes known as "deep breathing," has been shown to be effective in lowering levels of tension and anxiety. Since it can be done at any location and at any time, this method is a practical and easy approach to deal with stress and anxiety at any point in the day. Finding a quiet area to sit or lay down and focusing your attention on your breath while taking slow, deep breaths in through your nose and out through your mouth is the first step in developing the skill of practicing deep breathing.

Exercise:
The release of endorphins, which are naturally occurring chemicals that improve mood, is one of the primary benefits of physical activity for stress management and anxiety reduction. In addition, exercise may aid to enhance circulation, lower blood pressure, and general health, all of which can contribute to an improvement in kidney health. When beginning a new workout routine, it is essential to discuss the matter with a qualified medical professional, particularly if you suffer from renal illness.

Cognitive-behavioral therapy:
Cognitive-behavioral therapy, sometimes known as CBT, is a kind of talk therapy that focuses on

recognizing destructive thinking patterns and actions and working to alter such patterns. By encouraging more optimistic thought patterns and more physically active ways to deal with stressful situations, cognitive behavioral therapy (CBT) may be an efficient method for managing stress and anxiety. CBT may be conducted in a one-on-one setting with a therapist or in a group setting with several participants.

Social support:
Having a strong social support network is an important component of a successful stress and anxiety management strategy. By offering a sense of connection and purpose, activities such as talking with friends and family members, joining a support group, or volunteering may all assist in the reduction of feelings of stress and anxiety.

In conclusion, the consequences of stress and worry may be detrimental to our physical as well as mental health, including the health of our kidneys. Yet, there are a variety of strategies that can be used to take control of one's stress and anxiety levels, which, in turn, may assist to enhance one's kidney health. Techniques such as mindfulness meditation, yoga, progressive muscle relaxation, deep breathing, exercise, cognitive behavioral therapy, and social support are all useful tools for reducing anxiety and stress. Finding the method, or the combination of methods, that works the best for you is essential, and it is as essential to put that method, or those methods, into regular practice in order to experience the rewards.

Improving mental health and well-being

Enhancing one's emotional and overall physical well-being may have a beneficial effect on one's kidney health. Research have indicated that people who have chronic kidney disease (CKD) have a greater chance of developing mental health conditions such as depression and anxiety, both of which may have a severe impact on an individual's overall health as well as their quality of life. On the other hand, improvements in a person's mental health and well-being may have a positive impact on their overall health outcomes when they have renal disease.

One of the ways that enhancing one's mental health may have a favorable influence on one's kidney function is by lowering one's overall level of stress. Prolonged stress may have harmful consequences on the body, including elevated blood pressure, inflammation, and reduced immunological function. All of these factors can contribute to the development and progression of kidney disease. Chronic stress can be avoided by reducing your stress levels. Individuals may be able to lessen the adverse effects of stress on their kidneys if they lower their overall stress levels through methods such as meditation, yoga, or therapy.

Enhancing one's mental health and sense of well-being may also contribute to improved adherence to the treatment regimens prescribed for renal disease. Those who struggle with depression and anxiety may find it more challenging to adhere to their pharmaceutical regimen, keep their scheduled visits, and implement other necessary lifestyle adjustments. Those who work to improve their mental health may find that they are more motivated to manage their renal illness and are more able to do so. This may allow them to make good improvements to their health.

Enhancing one's mental health may also result in the adoption of healthy lifestyle habits, which in turn can have a beneficial effect on one's renal health. For instance, people who are battling mental health conditions such as depression or anxiety may be more inclined to engage in activities that are detrimental to their health, such as smoking, drinking alcohol, or having a bad diet. It is possible that persons who improve their mental health will be more inclined to adopt better choices, which in turn may lessen the chance of developing renal disease.

It is also important to note that patients with renal disease may see an improvement in their quality of life if they work to improve their mental health. Having kidney disease may be a difficult and frequently stressful condition; however, taking steps to improve mental health and well-being can assist people in coping with the emotional and physical demands that come along with having the illness. This has the potential to result in improved results for one's overall health as well as an increase in one's quality of life.

To summarize, enhancing one's mental health and overall well-being may have a beneficial effect on one's renal health. Individuals with kidney disease may be able to improve their overall health outcomes and their ability to manage their condition by lowering their levels of stress, increasing their adherence to treatment regimens, adopting healthier lifestyle choices, and improving their overall quality of life. It is essential for persons who have renal disease to place a high priority on their mental health and to look for appropriate assistance and therapy if it is required.

Chapter 8: Preventing Kidney Disease

Steps to prevent kidney disease

Kidney disease is a severe and persistent disorder that impacts the lives of millions of individuals all over the globe. There are a number of things a person may do to lower their chance of having kidney disease; but, there are some aspects of their health that cannot be changed, such as their age, their genetics, and any preexisting medical disorders. These stages are as follows:

- A healthy weight should be maintained. Being obese or overweight raises the risk of having kidney disease because it increases the likelihood of acquiring high blood pressure and diabetes. Keeping a healthy weight via a combination of a nutritious food and consistent physical activity is essential in the fight against kidney disease.

- Frequent exercise may help avoid high blood pressure and diabetes, two of the primary causes of kidney disease. Regular exercise can help prevent high blood pressure and diabetes. In addition to this, it assists in the maintenance of a healthy weight, which is essential in lowering the chance of developing renal disease.

- Diabetes, the leading cause of kidney damage, may be managed by maintaining healthy blood sugar levels. Individuals who have diabetes should have a tight relationship with their healthcare professionals in order to effectively regulate their blood sugar levels and stave off consequences like kidney damage.

- Take care of your blood pressure: prolonged exposure to high blood pressure might lead to kidney injury. Kidney disease may be avoided by maintaining a healthy blood pressure level, which can be done by medication and regular monitoring of blood pressure levels.

- Put out that cigarette! Smoking is a risk factor for a wide variety of health disorders, including renal disease, so if you do it, put it out! Putting down the cigarette may help lower one's chances of developing renal disease as well as other health problems.

- Reduce your use of alcohol since drinking too much may harm your kidneys over time. Consuming alcohol in moderation may be helpful in warding against renal disease.

- Maintaining proper hydration is essential, since kidney damage may be avoided by draining harmful toxins out of the body, which can be accomplished by drinking enough of water. It is essential to drink enough of water throughout the day, but this is particularly true when the temperature is high or when you are participating in strenuous activities.

- Take caution not to overindulge in non-prescription pain relievers: When used in excessive amounts, nonsteroidal anti-inflammatory medicines (NSAIDs) like ibuprofen may cause long-term harm to the kidneys. It is essential to take these drugs exactly as advised and to consult a medical professional prior to beginning a treatment regimen that involves their use.

- Test your kidney function on a frequent basis. If kidney disease is detected at an early stage, when it is simpler to treat, regular renal function testing may assist. Individuals who have a history of renal disease in their family or who have other risk factors should get their kidney function checked on a regular basis.

- Have a healthy diet: Eating a diet that is both balanced and rich in nutrients may help avoid kidney disease. This is accomplished by lowering the chance of developing diabetes and high blood pressure. It is advisable to have a diet that is abundant in fruits, vegetables, cereals that are whole, and sources of lean protein.

To summarize, prevention is the most important factor in lowering the chance of developing renal disease. Individuals may safeguard their kidney health by taking preventative measures such as leading a healthy lifestyle and keeping a close eye on any pre-existing diseases they may have. It is essential to design a specialized preventative strategy for kidney disease in close collaboration with a healthcare specialist if you want the best results.

Screening and early detection

The prevention of kidney disease relies heavily on screening tests and spotting problems in their earliest stages. There is a good chance that kidney disease will not present any symptoms in the majority of patients until the illness has proceeded to an advanced stage. Kidney disease may be slowed or even stopped in its tracks if it is diagnosed and treated in its early stages, which leads to better overall results and a lower risk of complications.

Screening tests, such as those performed on the blood and the urine, are able to identify indicators of kidney disease even before the symptoms manifest themselves. Those who are at a greater risk of developing kidney disease, such as those who have diabetes, high blood pressure, or a history of renal disease in their families, should get routine screenings.

When kidney disease is identified at an earlier stage, medical professionals are better able to collaborate with patients to devise a treatment strategy. This strategy may involve making adjustments to the patient's way of life, taking medications, or engaging in some other form of intervention in order to halt or slow the progression of the disease. This may assist in reducing the risk of consequences such as renal failure, cardiovascular disease, and other health issues connected to kidney disease.

In addition, early identification of kidney disease enables better treatment of underlying disorders, such as diabetes and high blood pressure, which may contribute to the progression of renal disease. Individuals may lower their chance of acquiring kidney disease or halt the advancement of the illness by successfully treating the factors that put them at risk.

In conclusion, screening tests and being diagnosed at an early stage are both very important in the fight against kidney disease. When kidney illness is detected in its earliest stages, medical professionals are better able to collaborate with patients to devise appropriate treatment regimens that may delay or arrest the advancement of the disease. This ultimately leads to better results and a lower risk of complications. It is recommended that people who are at an increased risk of developing kidney disease undergo routine screenings, and it is essential to treat the underlying conditions that contribute to the development of kidney disease in order to lower the risk of developing this potentially debilitating condition.

Managing underlying health conditions

Managing underlying health conditions is crucial for preventing and slowing the progression of kidney disease. Certain health conditions can damage the kidneys, including high blood pressure, diabetes, and heart disease. Proper management of these conditions can help to protect the kidneys and prevent further damage.

High Blood Pressure: High blood pressure, also known as hypertension, is one of the leading causes of kidney disease. Over time, high blood pressure can damage the small blood vessels in the kidneys, making it harder for them to filter waste and fluid from the blood. This can lead to kidney disease and even kidney failure.

To manage high blood pressure and protect the kidneys, lifestyle changes and medications may be necessary. Lifestyle changes can include:

- Eating a healthy diet low in sodium and high in fruits and vegetables
- Getting regular exercise
- Maintaining a healthy weight
- Limiting alcohol consumption
- Quitting smoking
- Reducing stress

Medications may also be necessary to manage high blood pressure, including angiotensin-converting enzyme (ACE) inhibitors and angiotensin II receptor blockers (ARBs). These medications can help to relax the blood vessels and lower blood pressure, which can protect the kidneys from damage.

Diabetes: Diabetes is another leading cause of kidney disease. High levels of glucose in the blood can damage the small blood vessels in the kidneys, reducing their ability to filter waste and fluid from the blood.

To manage diabetes and protect the kidneys, lifestyle changes and medications may be necessary. Lifestyle changes can include:

- Eating a healthy diet low in sugar and high in fiber
- Getting regular exercise
- Monitoring blood glucose levels
- Maintaining a healthy weight
- Limiting alcohol consumption
- Quitting smoking
- Reducing stress

Medications may also be necessary to manage diabetes, including insulin and oral medications such as metformin. These medications can help to lower blood glucose levels and reduce the risk of kidney damage.

Heart Disease: Heart disease is also a risk factor for kidney disease. Atherosclerosis, or the hardening and narrowing of the arteries, can reduce blood flow to the kidneys, making it harder for them to filter waste and fluid from the blood.

To manage heart disease and protect the kidneys, lifestyle changes and medications may be necessary. Lifestyle changes can include:

- Eating a healthy diet low in saturated and trans fats
- Getting regular exercise
- Maintaining a healthy weight
- Limiting alcohol consumption
- Quitting smoking
- Reducing stress

Medications may also be necessary to manage heart disease, including cholesterol-lowering medications such as statins and blood-thinning medications such as aspirin. These medications can help to reduce the risk of atherosclerosis and protect the kidneys from damage.

Overall, managing underlying health conditions is crucial for preventing and slowing the progression of kidney disease. By making lifestyle changes and taking necessary medications, individuals can protect their kidneys and maintain their overall health. It is important to work with a healthcare provider to develop a plan that is tailored to individual needs and conditions.

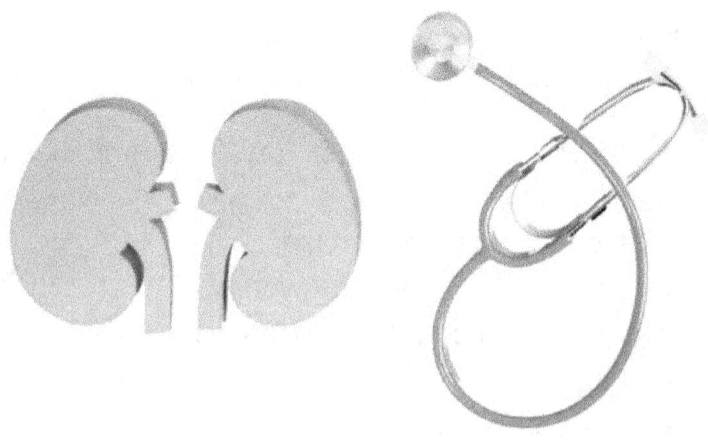

Chapter 9: Importance of Nutrition in Reversing Kidney Disease

Key nutrients and vitamins that support kidney health

A healthy diet is one of the most important factors in maintaining kidney function and may even play a role in the reversal of renal disease. To be more specific, there are a number of essential minerals and vitamins that are vital for maintaining healthy kidneys. The following is a list of some of the most important minerals and vitamins that may promote healthy kidney function:

Protein: Protein is an important ingredient that helps the body develop and repair tissues. Protein may be found in meat, fish, eggs, and dairy products. Nonetheless, it is essential for persons who have renal illness to carefully regulate their consumption of protein, since an excessive amount of protein may put stress on the kidneys. A dietitian may assist in determining the correct quantity of protein to ingest depending on an individual's specific requirements as well as the functioning of their kidneys.

Potassium: Potassium is a mineral that plays an important role in the body's ability to maintain proper fluid balance and blood pressure. Hyperkalemia is a condition that may be harmful for those who already have renal disease. High amounts of potassium in the blood. As a result, it is essential to keep track of the amount of potassium consumed and to adhere to a diet that is low in potassium. This may require cutting down on certain fruits and vegetables.

Phosphorus: Phosphorus is a mineral that assists in the formation and repair of bones and teeth, in addition to assisting in the transformation of food into energy for the body. Having high amounts of phosphorus in the blood, also known as hyperphosphatemia, may lead to issues with the bones and the heart in patients who already have renal disease. Because of this, it is essential to keep a close eye on the amount of phosphorus that one consumes and to adhere to a diet that is low in phosphorus. This may include cutting down on certain types of dairy products, meats, and processed foods.

Calcium: Calcium is a mineral that helps regulate muscle and nerve function, in addition to being essential for maintaining healthy bones. Calcium levels in the blood might become unbalanced and abnormal in patients who suffer from renal disease. It is essential to keep track of the amount of calcium that one consumes, to adhere to a diet that contains an appropriate amount of both calcium and phosphorus, and to take any supplements that have been prescribed by a medical professional.

Vitamin D: Absorption of calcium in the body is facilitated by vitamin D, which also contributes to overall bone health. Those who have renal illness are more likely to have vitamin D levels that are out of whack, which may lead to bone issues. It is essential to keep track of vitamin D levels and to take any supplements that have been prescribed to you by a medical professional.

Iron: Iron is a mineral that plays an important role in the production of red blood cells as well as the delivery of oxygen to the body's tissues. An iron imbalance may develop in patients with renal illness, which can ultimately result in the development of anemia. It is essential to keep track of iron levels and consume a diet that is abundant in iron. Some examples of iron-rich foods are lean meats, beans, and dark green leafy vegetables.

<u>B vitamins</u>: The B vitamins, which include thiamin, riboflavin, niacin, and vitamin B6, are essential for the production of red blood cells, the maintenance of good neuronal function, and the conversion of food into usable energy. It is possible for the levels of B vitamins to become unbalanced when a person has renal illness. It is essential to keep track of your B vitamin levels and take any supplements that have been prescribed to you by a medical professional.

In general, eating a diet that is both well-balanced and rich in nutrients is essential for promoting healthy kidney function and may be of assistance in reversing renal disease. Working with a nutritionist or another source of healthcare may assist ensure that nutritional demands are satisfied and that the diet is customized to the individual's needs as well as their kidney function.

Foods to avoid for kidney health

It is very important to eat healthily in order to keep your kidneys in good condition, and there are certain foods that should be avoided in order to either stop or slow the progression of kidney disease. Avoiding these meals can help you stay healthy:

<u>Processed and packaged foods</u>: Processed and packaged foods often include a high amount of salt, as well as preservatives and additives, all of which may be damaging to the kidneys. Chips, crackers, canned soups and veggies, frozen dinners, and deli meats are some examples of the goods that fall into this category.

<u>Red Meat</u>: Since it has a high percentage of protein, red meat might make the kidneys have to work harder. In addition to this, it has a high phosphorus content, which might make it challenging for persons with renal illness to clear the substance from their bodies.

<u>Dairy products</u>: Products made from milk and other sources of dairy include significant quantities of phosphorus and calcium, two minerals that are known to be detrimental to kidney health. Individuals who have renal illness should cut down on their use of dairy products or look for alternatives that are lower in phosphorus.

Sodium: Excess sodium may lead to a rise in blood pressure and can also be harmful to the kidneys. Those who suffer from renal illness have to restrict their salt consumption to fewer than 2,300 milligrams per day.

Sugary drinks: Beverages high in sugar, such as soda and energy drinks, have been shown to raise blood pressure and cause damage to the kidneys. Individuals who have renal illness have to steer clear of sugary drinks and choose instead for water or beverages that are not sweetened.

Alcohol: Consuming alcohol may lead to a rise in blood pressure as well as renal damage. Those who have renal illness should cut down significantly on their alcohol use or abstain entirely.

It is essential to see a healthcare physician or a qualified dietitian in order to get individualized dietary advice that are derived from one's specific requirements and medical history.

Tips for planning a kidney-friendly diet

Planning a kidney-friendly diet can be a challenging task, especially if you are new to managing kidney disease. However, with a few tips and strategies, it is possible to create a healthy and satisfying diet that supports your kidney health.

Here are some tips for planning a kidney-friendly diet:

- Consult with a dietitian: A registered dietitian who specializes in kidney disease can help you create a personalized meal plan that meets your specific dietary needs. They can also help you understand which foods to avoid and which ones to incorporate into your diet.
- Limit sodium: Sodium can increase blood pressure and put stress on the kidneys. Limiting sodium intake to less than 2,300 mg per day can help to reduce the risk of kidney damage. Avoid adding salt to your food and choose fresh or frozen foods instead of processed or canned foods, which are often high in sodium.
- Choose kidney-friendly protein sources: Protein is essential for maintaining muscle mass and overall health, but excessive protein intake can be harmful to the kidneys. Choosing high-quality protein sources that are easy on the kidneys, such as fish, poultry,

eggs, and low-fat dairy products, can help to maintain kidney health.

- Control phosphorus intake: High levels of phosphorus in the blood can lead to bone and heart problems. Limiting phosphorus intake to less than 1,000 mg per day can help to manage kidney disease. Foods high in phosphorus include dairy products, nuts, beans, and whole grains.

- Monitor potassium intake: Potassium is important for muscle and heart function, but high levels can be dangerous for people with kidney disease. The recommended intake of potassium for people with kidney disease varies based on individual needs. Foods high in potassium include bananas, oranges, potatoes, spinach, and tomatoes.

- Choose healthy fats: Healthy fats, such as those found in nuts, seeds, and fatty fish, can help to reduce inflammation and protect the kidneys. Limiting saturated and trans fats found in processed and fried foods can also help to protect kidney health.

- Stay hydrated: Staying hydrated is essential for kidney health. Drinking enough water and other fluids can help to flush out toxins and waste products, reducing the risk of kidney damage.

- Consider vitamin and mineral supplements: People with kidney disease may have difficulty getting enough vitamins and minerals from their diet. Your healthcare provider or dietitian can help you determine if you need supplements and which ones to take.

By following these tips and working with a healthcare provider or dietitian, you can create a kidney-friendly diet that supports your overall health and helps to manage kidney disease.

Recipes for reversing kidney disease

Eating the correct foods will surely help you in reversing kidney diseases.

Here are some general guidelines for creating kidney-friendly meals:

- Choose low-sodium foods: Sodium can increase blood pressure and put a strain on the kidneys. Aim to limit your sodium intake to 1,500-2,300 mg per day.
- Include lean protein: Good sources of protein for people with kidney disease include chicken, fish, eggs, and tofu. Avoid high-

protein diets and limit intake of red meat, which can increase the workload on the kidneys.

- Increase intake of fruits and vegetables: Fruits and vegetables are packed with vitamins and minerals that are important for kidney health. Choose low-potassium options such as berries, apples, and green beans.
- Choose whole grains: Whole grains are high in fiber and nutrients, and can help regulate blood sugar levels. Good options include brown rice, quinoa, and whole-wheat bread.
- Limit phosphorus: People with kidney disease may need to limit their intake of phosphorus, which can build up in the body and cause bone and heart problems. Avoid processed foods and limit intake of dairy products.

Here are some recipe ideas for kidney-friendly meals:

Breakfast:
- Omelette with low-fat cheese, spinach, and mushrooms
- Steel-cut oatmeal with blueberries and almonds

- Whole-grain toast with almond butter and sliced banana

Lunch:
- Tuna salad with low-fat mayo, celery, and carrots on whole-wheat bread
- Spinach salad with grilled chicken, strawberries, and balsamic vinaigrette
- Black bean soup with a side of steamed green beans

Dinner:
- Baked salmon with lemon, garlic, and herbs, served with roasted asparagus and quinoa
- Stir-fry with tofu, broccoli, bell peppers, and brown rice
- Turkey chili with kidney beans, diced tomatoes, and spices

Snacks:
- Apple slices with almond butter
- Carrot sticks with hummus
- Greek yogurt with berries and chopped nuts

It's important to remember that everyone's nutritional needs are different and that these are general guidelines. Consult with a registered dietitian for personalized advice on creating a kidney-friendly diet.

Two-week meal plan

Here is the complete two-week meal plan for reversing kidney disease:

Week 1:

Monday:
- Breakfast: Oatmeal with blueberries and a boiled egg
- Snack: Sliced apple with almond butter
- Lunch: Turkey and cheese wrap with a side of raw carrots and celery
- Snack: Small handful of unsalted mixed nuts
- Dinner: Baked salmon with roasted asparagus and quinoa

Tuesday:
- Breakfast: Greek yogurt with sliced peaches and a hard-boiled egg
- Snack: Baby carrots with hummus
- Lunch: Grilled chicken salad with mixed greens, cherry tomatoes, and cucumber
- Snack: Small apple with string cheese

- Dinner: Lentil soup with a side of steamed broccoli

Wednesday:
- Breakfast: Scrambled eggs with spinach and a whole-grain English muffin
- Snack: Sliced cucumber with tzatziki dip
- Lunch: Tuna salad with mixed greens, tomato, and cucumber
- Snack: Small handful of unsalted mixed nuts
- Dinner: Baked chicken breast with roasted Brussels sprouts and brown rice

Thursday:
- Breakfast: Whole-grain toast with avocado and a hard-boiled egg
- Snack: Sliced apple with almond butter
- Lunch: Veggie burger with a side of roasted sweet potatoes
- Snack: Baby carrots with hummus
- Dinner: Grilled steak with roasted zucchini and quinoa

Friday:
- Breakfast: Greek yogurt with mixed berries and a boiled egg
- Snack: Sliced cucumber with tzatziki dip

- Lunch: Chicken and vegetable stir-fry with brown rice
- Snack: Small apple with string cheese
- Dinner: Baked salmon with roasted asparagus and sweet potato fries

Saturday:
- Breakfast: Whole-grain waffles with mixed berries and a hard-boiled egg
- Snack: Sliced bell peppers with hummus
- Lunch: Quinoa salad with mixed greens, cherry tomatoes, and cucumber
- Snack: Small handful of unsalted mixed nuts
- Dinner: Baked chicken breast with roasted Brussels sprouts and brown rice

Sunday:
- Breakfast: Omelette with spinach and mushrooms and a whole-grain English muffin
- Snack: Sliced apple with almond butter
- Lunch: Turkey and cheese wrap with a side of raw carrots and celery
- Snack: Baby carrots with hummus
- Dinner: Beef and vegetable stew with a side of steamed broccoli

Week 2:

Monday:

- Breakfast: Greek yogurt with mixed berries and a hard-boiled egg
- Snack: Sliced cucumber with tzatziki dip
- Lunch: Lentil soup with a side of steamed broccoli
- Snack: Small apple with string cheese
- Dinner: Baked chicken breast with roasted Brussels sprouts and brown rice

Tuesday:

- Breakfast: Omelette with spinach and mushrooms and a whole-grain English muffin
- Snack: Sliced apple with almond butter
- Lunch: Grilled chicken salad with mixed greens, cherry tomatoes, and cucumber
- Snack: Small handful of unsalted mixed nuts
- Dinner: Baked salmon with roasted asparagus and sweet potato fries

Wednesday:

- Breakfast: Whole-grain toast with avocado and a hard-boiled egg
- Snack: Baby carrots with hummus
- Lunch: Turkey and cheese wrap with a side of raw carrots and celery
- Snack: Sliced bell peppers with hummus

- Dinner: Beef and vegetable stew with a side of steamed broccoli

Thursday:
- Breakfast: Greek yogurt with sliced peaches and a hard-boiled egg
- Snack: Sliced apple with almond butter
- Lunch: Tuna salad made with canned tuna, low-fat mayonnaise, diced celery and onion, served with whole wheat crackers and carrot sticks
- Snack: Small serving of unsalted popcorn
- Dinner: Baked chicken breast with roasted vegetables (carrots, bell peppers, zucchini) and a side salad with mixed greens, cherry tomatoes, and low-fat vinaigrette dressing

Friday:
- Breakfast: Oatmeal cooked with low-fat milk, topped with sliced banana and chopped walnuts
- Snack: Low-sodium string cheese with whole grain crackers
- Lunch: Grilled salmon with roasted asparagus and a side of quinoa salad (quinoa, diced tomatoes, diced cucumbers, and lemon vinaigrette)
- Snack: Carrot sticks with hummus

- Dinner: Beef stir-fry with mixed vegetables (broccoli, bell peppers, onion) and brown rice

Saturday:
- Breakfast: Scrambled eggs with spinach and mushrooms, served with a slice of whole wheat toast
- Snack: Small serving of fresh berries
- Lunch: Turkey and cheese sandwich on whole wheat bread with a side of vegetable soup (low sodium)
- Snack: Plain Greek yogurt with a drizzle of honey and chopped nuts
- Dinner: Grilled chicken kabobs with cherry tomatoes, onions, and bell peppers, served with a side of brown rice and a mixed greens salad with low-fat dressing

Sunday:
- Breakfast: Whole grain waffles with fresh berries and a dollop of plain Greek yogurt
- Snack: Low-sodium beef jerky with unsalted almonds
- Lunch: Vegetable and bean chili with a side of whole grain crackers and a side salad with mixed greens, cherry tomatoes, and low-fat vinaigrette dressing
- Snack: Sliced cucumber with hummus

- Dinner: Grilled shrimp with roasted broccoli and a side of wild rice

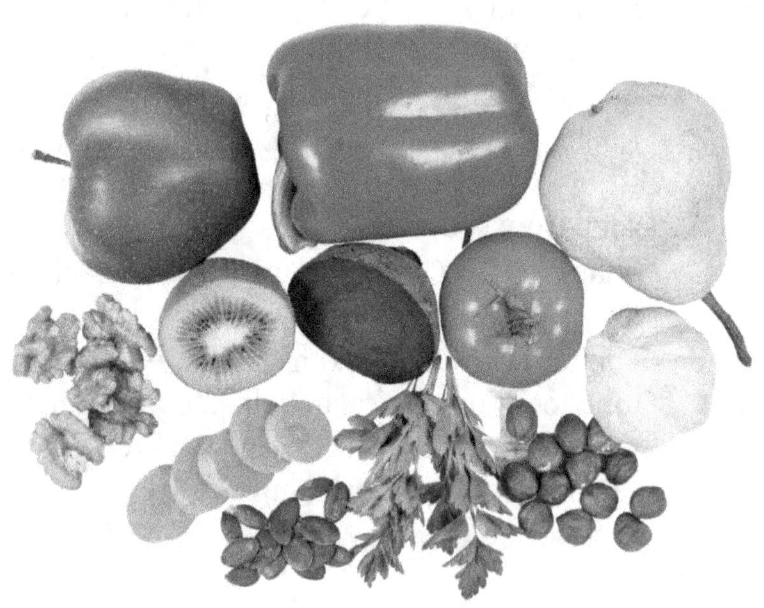

Chapter 9: Case Studies and Success Stories

Real-life examples of people who have successfully reversed kidney disease

There are numerous real-life examples of people who have successfully reversed kidney disease through lifestyle changes and medical treatment. Here are a few examples:

<u>Mary's Story:</u>
Mary was diagnosed with stage 3 chronic kidney disease and was devastated by the news. She had struggled with her health for many years, and the thought of kidney failure and dialysis was overwhelming. Mary knew she needed to make a change, and her nephrologist recommended a kidney-friendly diet.

At first, Mary struggled to adjust to the new way of eating, but with the help of a registered dietitian, she slowly began to incorporate more kidney-friendly foods into her diet. She focused on lean proteins, such as chicken and fish, and limited her intake of high-sodium and high-potassium foods.

As Mary's health improved, she began to feel more energetic and vibrant. She was no longer in constant pain, and her kidney function had improved significantly. Mary was able to avoid dialysis and continued to live a healthy, active lifestyle.

<u>John's Story:</u>
John had been living with type 2 diabetes for many years, and as a result, he had developed chronic kidney disease. He was struggling to manage his blood sugar and his kidney function continued to decline. John knew he needed to make a change, but he wasn't sure where to start.

With the help of his healthcare team, John began to incorporate more plant-based foods into his diet, such as whole grains, fruits, and vegetables. He also cut back on processed foods, sugar, and salt.

As John's diet improved, his blood sugar and blood pressure began to stabilize, and his kidney function improved. He was no longer in constant pain, and he felt more energized and alive than he had in years. John's story shows that even small dietary changes can have a significant impact on kidney health.

<u>Sarah's Story:</u>
Sarah had been struggling with kidney disease for many years, and despite her best efforts, her kidney function continued to decline. She was tired of feeling sick and tired, and she knew she needed to make a change.

Sarah began working with a registered dietitian who specialized in kidney health. Together, they developed a meal plan that focused on nutrient-dense foods, such as lean proteins, whole grains, and vegetables. Sarah also made a conscious effort to stay hydrated by drinking plenty of water throughout the day.

As Sarah's diet improved, she began to feel more energized and focused. Her kidney function improved, and she was able to avoid dialysis. Sarah's story shows that with dedication and hard work, it is possible to reverse kidney disease and improve overall health.

These are just a few examples of how people have successfully reversed kidney disease. It's important to note that every individual's situation is unique, and what works for one person may not work for another. It's important to work closely with a healthcare provider to develop a personalized treatment plan for managing kidney disease.

Strategies and lifestyle changes that helped them improve kidney function

The three case studies of persons who were able to effectively reverse renal disease by making adjustments to their lifestyles indicate the efficacy of adopting a healthy lifestyle in restoring kidney function. [Case studies] These people made major adjustments to their dietary habits and their levels of physical activity, in addition to making steps to better manage their stress and receive sufficient amounts of restful sleep.

One of the most important things that they did was to concentrate on eating a kidney-friendly diet. This involved decreasing the amount of processed and high-sodium foods that they consumed while simultaneously increasing the amount of fresh fruits and vegetables, sources of lean protein, and whole grains that they consumed. In addition to this, they made an attempt to maintain proper hydration by consuming a sufficient amount of water and reducing the amount of sugary drinks they consumed.

Walking, cycling, and swimming were just some of the examples of everyday physical activities that all three people included in their schedules on a consistent basis. They were able to control their weight, lower their levels of stress, and enhance their general health by engaging in activities that required physical movement.

Meditation, yoga, and other similar activities, as well as workouts that focus on deep breathing, were some of the methods that they used to help them better deal with stress. They were able to enhance their mental and emotional well-being, which in turn helped to decrease inflammation and supported the health of their kidneys. This was achieved by lowering their overall stress levels.

Last but not least, they made an effort to give sleep and relaxation a higher priority, realizing that having an adequate amount of restful sleep is critical to maintaining overall health and fitness. They were able to enhance the quality of their sleep and promote their general health by adopting adjustments to their typical pattern of sleeping, such as maintaining a consistent bedtime and refraining from consuming coffee in the evenings.

Overall, these three people were able to effectively reverse renal disease by adopting a healthy lifestyle that focused on a kidney-friendly diet, regular physical exercise, stress management, and appropriate restful sleep. This allowed them to achieve the desired result. These tactics not only made them feel better physically and psychologically, but they also restored their kidney function, which gave them a new lease on life.

Challenges and obstacles they faced along the way

In the process of reversing kidney disease, there are often challenges and obstacles that people face. The three real-life examples mentioned earlier have also faced their fair share of difficulties along the way.

In the case of John, one of the main challenges he faced was his love for unhealthy foods such as fast food and processed snacks. He found it challenging to give up these foods and adjust to a kidney-friendly diet. In addition, he struggled with maintaining a regular exercise routine, as he found it difficult to balance work and his new lifestyle changes. However, John's determination to improve his health and the support of his family and healthcare team helped him overcome these challenges and stay on track with his kidney-friendly diet and exercise routine.

For Sarah, the main obstacle was the emotional toll of living with kidney disease. She struggled with anxiety and depression, and found it challenging to adjust to the physical limitations that came with her condition. However, through counseling and support from her healthcare team and loved ones, she was able to manage her mental health and stay motivated in her journey towards better kidney function.

Similarly, Marry faced many challenges along the way. She struggled with the changes to her diet and found it difficult to resist her old favorite foods. She also experienced physical symptoms, such as headaches and fatigue, as her body adjusted to the new diet. Additionally, she found it challenging to make time for exercise and self-care while juggling work and family responsibilities. Despite these obstacles, Marry remained committed to her health and continued to make progress towards improving her kidney function. She found support from her healthcare team and her family, who encouraged her to stay on track and reminded her of her goals. With time, Marry was able to incorporate these lifestyle changes into her daily routine and regain control over her health.

Overall, the journey to reversing kidney disease can be challenging, but with the right support and strategies in place, it is possible to overcome obstacles and achieve improved kidney function.

Lessons learned and advice for others on the same journey

The stories of Sarah, Marry and John show us that it is possible to reverse kidney disease through lifestyle changes and diet modifications. Here are some key lessons and advice that can be taken from their experiences:

- Education and knowledge are critical. Understanding the causes and symptoms of kidney disease, as well as the steps needed to reverse it, is essential. Research and learn about kidney disease, and work with healthcare professionals to create a plan tailored to your specific needs.
- Diet and nutrition play a significant role. Eating a balanced and healthy diet, with the right amounts of protein, carbohydrates, and healthy fats, is essential for kidney health. Restricting salt and other harmful substances is also crucial. Consult with a registered

dietitian who specializes in kidney disease to get a tailored diet plan.

- Regular exercise and physical activity are key. Exercise can help to manage weight, lower blood pressure, and reduce stress levels, which are all factors that contribute to kidney disease.
- Medications and treatment may be necessary. In some cases, medication may be required to treat underlying conditions such as high blood pressure or diabetes. Following medical advice and taking medications as prescribed is essential.
- Lifestyle changes require discipline and commitment. Changing habits can be difficult, but it is essential to maintain a consistent and disciplined approach to ensure that lifestyle changes become permanent. Celebrate small successes along the way to stay motivated.
- Support from family and friends is crucial. The journey to reversing kidney disease can be challenging and lonely. Surrounding oneself with family and friends who provide support, encouragement, and motivation can be very helpful.

In conclusion, the stories of Sarah, Marry and John illustrate that it is possible to reverse kidney disease through lifestyle changes and diet modifications. It requires commitment, discipline, and a willingness to learn and make changes, but the rewards of better health and well-being are well worth the effort.

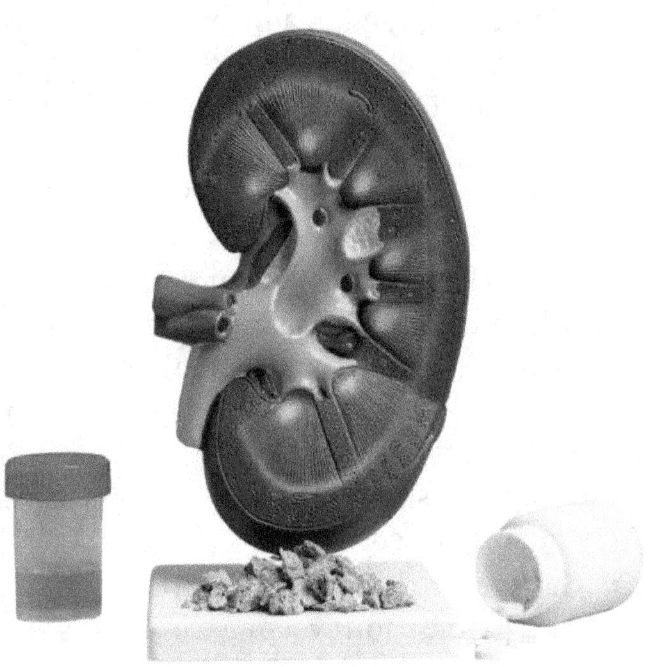

Chapter 10: Conclusion

The importance of kidney health

In conclusion, maintaining good kidney health is of the utmost significance since the kidneys play an essential part in the body's ability to operate normally. The kidneys are responsible for removing waste products and excess fluid from the blood, controlling blood pressure, producing hormones, and contributing to the maintenance of the acid-base balance in the body. Kidney disease is a dangerous disorder that may lead to a broad variety of problems, including renal failure and cardiovascular disease. Kidney disease is a leading cause of death in the United States.

Thankfully, there are a lot of things you can do to keep your kidneys in good condition and even enhance them. Regular exercise, the management of stress, avoiding dangerous drugs such as cigarettes and excessive alcohol use, and controlling underlying health disorders such as diabetes and high blood pressure are all things that may help prevent and manage kidney disease.

A diet that is kidney-friendly consists of meals that are low in sodium, low in phosphorus, and low in potassium, but that nevertheless provide an acceptable amount of protein and the important nutrients. Nutrition is another vital component in maintaining healthy kidneys. In addition, several essential minerals and vitamins, including omega-3 fatty acids, vitamin D, and iron, have been demonstrated to promote kidney health and may be integrated into a balanced diet. These nutrients and vitamins have been proved to be beneficial to kidney health.

The ability to diagnose and test for kidney illness early may also dramatically improve patient outcomes. This is because rapid treatment can either slow down or even stop the course of the disease. It is important to consult with a healthcare provider and to undergo regular screenings, particularly if you have risk factors such as a family history of kidney disease or underlying health conditions. In particular, it is important to consult with a healthcare provider if you have risk factors such as a family history of kidney disease.

In general, taking care of the health of your kidneys is a crucial component of maintaining both overall health and well-being for yourself. You may lower your chance of developing kidney disease and improve the outcomes of your condition if you are already living with kidney disease by adopting some positive adjustments to your lifestyle, such as following a healthy diet and getting frequent check-ups.

How to maintain healthy kidneys

It is essential for one's general health and well-being to take care of their kidneys and keep them in good shape. Individuals have a number of options at their disposal for maintaining healthy kidneys and warding off renal disease, including the following:

- Maintaining optimum hydration by consuming a sufficient amount of water and other fluids is essential for maintaining healthy kidney function. It is suggested that a person consumes at least 8 glasses of water on a daily basis.

- Consume a diet rich in fruits, vegetables, and whole grains. Eating a diet that is low in salt, sugar, and saturated fats while being high in these other food groups may help avoid kidney injury. Consuming a diet that is high in antioxidants is another way to help protect the kidneys from the harm that may be caused by free radicals.

- Regular exercise helps to maintain a healthy weight and reduce the risk of developing chronic diseases such as diabetes and high blood pressure, both of which are risk factors for kidney disease. Regular exercise also helps to reduce the risk of developing heart disease, which is another risk factor for kidney disease.

- Treat chronic illnesses: Patients who suffer from chronic disorders such as diabetes or high blood pressure should collaborate with their primary care physician to develop a treatment plan that will help them manage their symptoms and reduce the risk of kidney damage.

- Stay away from cigarettes and cut down on alcohol if you want to protect your kidneys from the long-term harm caused by smoking and drinking too much alcohol. Giving up smoking and cutting down on alcohol use are two steps that may help preserve the kidneys.

- Take steps to manage your stress: extended periods of stress are associated with an increased likelihood of acquiring chronic illnesses such as diabetes and high blood pressure, both of which are risk factors for kidney disease. It is possible to lower stress levels and protect the kidneys by regularly engaging in stress management practices such as meditation, yoga, and deep breathing exercises.

- Attend all of your routine checkups Going to all of your routine checkups with your healthcare provider will help diagnose kidney disease early on, when it is at its most curable stage. Those who have a history of renal disease in their family or who have other risk factors for kidney disease should discuss their risk with their healthcare practitioner and undergo kidney function testing on a regular basis.

In conclusion, ensuring that one's kidneys remain in good condition is critical to one's overall health and well-being. Individuals may lower their chance of getting kidney disease and preserve their kidneys from harm by following these measures in order.

Hope for reversing kidney disease

Although being told you have kidney disease might be distressing, keep in mind that there is treatment available that can reverse your condition. Several individuals have been able to effectively cure their kidney illness and restore their health by combining different medical therapies, changes to their lifestyle, and maintaining a good mental attitude.

Early diagnosis and therapy is one of the most important factors in any attempt to reverse renal disease. You may avoid more damage to your kidneys and even reverse some of the harm that has already been done to them if you monitor your kidney function and cooperate with your healthcare team to address any underlying health concerns.

Adopting a diet that is kidney-friendly is another key component. Such a diet consists of consuming a lot of fresh fruits and vegetables, sources of lean protein, and healthy fats. You may help your kidneys repair and perform more effectively by avoiding processed foods, excessive salt, and any other dietary triggers that might damage renal function. Examples of such triggers include diabetes and high blood pressure.

Alterations to one's diet are only one component in curing renal disease; regular exercise and effective methods of stress management are other important factors. The benefits of exercise include an increase in circulation, a decrease in inflammation, and general promotion of health and wellbeing. Yoga, meditation, and deep breathing are some examples of stress management strategies that have been shown to help decrease cortisol levels and reduce inflammation, both of which are beneficial to kidney function.

It is essential to keep in mind that reversing renal disease is not a fast cure and calls for attention and commitment in order to be successful. It is possible to reclaim your health and enhance your kidney function if you have the appropriate mentality, support from loved ones and healthcare experts, and a desire to make adjustments to your lifestyle.

It is also essential to keep in mind that the course that kidney disease takes in the life of every person is different, and that the pace at which and the degree to which kidney function improves may differ from one individual to the next. You may, however, take preventative measures toward correcting your kidney disease and attaining your health goals by concentrating on the aspects of your life that are within your control, such as your food, your level of physical activity, and how you deal with stress.

In conclusion, reversing renal disease and regaining your health are both feasible goals to pursue. You may overcome the problems of kidney illness and live a happy, healthy life by working with the healthcare professionals who are caring for you, making adjustments to your lifestyle, and adopting a positive mental attitude.

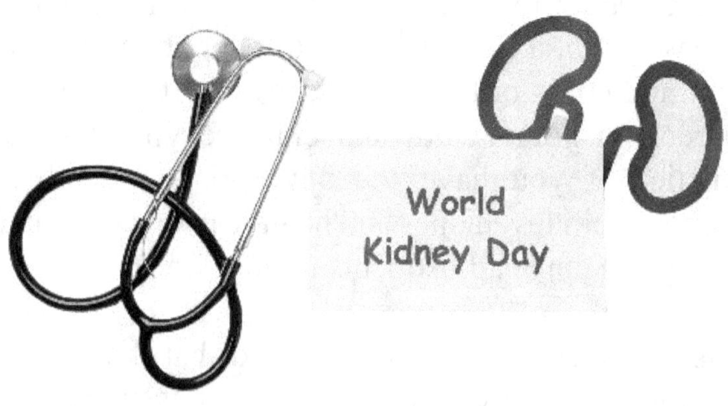

9 798387 108273